# NATURAL CHILDBIRTH IN MY LIFE

## Personal Accounts from Ignorance to Understanding

JULIE ANN YOUNG

Natural Childbirth - In My Life

Personal Accounts from Ignorance to Understanding

Copyright © Julie Ann Young

First published 2023

ISBN: 978-0-6458689-3-7 Paperback

ISBN: 978-0-6458689-4-4 E-Book

All rights reserved. Without limiting the rights under copyright reserved above, no part of this publication may be reproduced, stored in or introduced into a database and retrieval system or transmitted in any form or by any means (electronic, mechanical, photocopying, recording or otherwise) without the prior written permission of the owner of the copyright.

PLEASE BE AWARE descriptions of birthing events in this book may trigger past traumatic experiences.

Published with the assistance of Angel Key Publications
https://angelkey.com.au

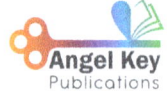

# CONTENTS

INTRODUCTION . . . . . . . . . . . . . . . . . . . . . . . . . . . V

*Chapter One*
Painful Ignorance Sets
Off a Learning Curve . . . . . . . . . . . . . . . . . . . . . . . . 1

*Chapter Two*
A Little Learning Went a Long Way. . . . . . . . . . . . . . . 25

*Chapter Three*
A BOOK REVIEW
"CHILDBIRTH WITHOUT FEAR" . . . . . . . . . . . . . . . . . . 39

*Chapter Four*
A BOOK REVIEW
"NO TIME FOR FEAR". . . . . . . . . . . . . . . . . . . . . . . . . 53

*Chapter Five*
Different Hospital –
Similar Stresses . . . . . . . . . . . . . . . . . . . . . . . . . . . 57

*Chapter Six*
A Very Difficult Lesson. . . . . . . . . . . . . . . . . . . . . . . 65

*Chapter Seven*
Homebirth . . . . . . . . . . . . . . . . . . . . . . . . . . . . . . . 73

# DEDICATION

*Dedicated with Love*

*To My 5 Children.*

*Mum*

# INTRODUCTION

Sharing our birth stories is now being seen as a way to empower women. Retelling a difficult story can help a mother to heal and telling positive stories can help to reduce fear. Women are being encouraged to talk more openly about their birthing experiences and their birth injuries.

For many years, I wanted to write my birth stories, but how could I do this without causing fear of childbirth? Finally, I came to the conclusion that I believe women, when educated and given full knowledge of the facts, are very capable of making their own decisions regardless of anything that had happened to me or anything that I might say.

In 1975, my first son and I had a very traumatic, hospital birth and I somehow knew that my ignorance had been a major contributing factor. Searching for a better experience the second time, I found a physiotherapist running antenatal classes near my home, so I joined up and this was the beginning of my acquiring some knowledge of childbirth. The method she taught followed the teachings of "Natural Childbirth" by Dr Grantly Dick-Read, although, at the time I didn't realise this.

Whilst I was able to walk this path, I am very much aware that there are women who, for many different reasons, and through no fault of their own, will need professional medical care to have their babies. Telling of my experiences is not meant to devalue the role of medical professionals in those instances.

This is not a text book on childbirth and I am not a healthcare professional. I'm writing as the mother of five children and I feel that in sharing my experiences, I can best explain how I found out about natural childbirth, and was able to practice its methods. At present, in my culture in Australia, childbirth largely belongs in the medical realm of hospitals with doctors and midwives in attendance, where mothers are "delivered".

After having four hospital births, I sought for the birth of my fifth child, a planned homebirth. But I may not have been able to do this without being in good health, becoming educated myself and having excellent care and support from a homebirth midwife, close family and friends.

After every birth, I always wrote down what I'd experienced. Among other occupations, from the age of 15 years, I had been a legal stenographer. It was easy for me to record my accounts. At the time, I didn't realise that this was also a form of catharsis, of releasing strong emotions. Some of my birthing experiences were joyful and some extremely painful, and I gathered knowledge from each one.

My experiences may bear no resemblance to any other mother's, in that we are all individuals and our needs and responses to people and circumstances can differ greatly. Yet, I now feel that every woman's birthing narrative is valuable. It provides the opportunity to share with other mothers and can be part of a healing process. It's taken me many years, but I've finally felt it is acceptable to write of my childbirth journeys and explain how I came to understand natural childbirth in my life.

*Julie Ann Young*
4th November 2023

*Chapter One*

# PAINFUL IGNORANCE SETS OFF A LEARNING CURVE

Largely due to a lack of education on the subject, the birth of my first child was a very painful experience. It was a forceps delivery, which in the light of other experience and knowledge, I now know was totally avoidable. In part, that is one of the main reasons for writing this book. My apologies to any reader who is disturbed by my description of events; it was a grim show for which I was unprepared, but I learned from my mistakes and those of others, and had some better times later on.

My childbirth history starts in Australia in 1974. At 27 years of age, I found out that I was pregnant with my first child. One of my friends was a registered midwife and I asked her whom I needed to see, she recommended the local obstetrician, as he was considered the very best in our neighbourhood. My husband and I had private health insurance and so I made an appointment.

At my first visit, this doctor gave me a very comprehensive examination. I needed to remove all my clothes and get under a sheet. He also did a smear test, which I'd never had before. I was fortunate to have no health problems. Visiting his surgery in the months that followed, it was often so busy there was standing room only. Sometimes after a long wait, they asked me to re-book and come back the next day. Knowing nothing, I was a very submissive patient and hardly asked any questions. Like many women at that time, I put all my trust and confidence in this doctor, because I thought he was the expert and I knew nothing, which was true.

From another friend, I found out that antenatal classes with a physiotherapist were being conducted, but you had to get a referral from the doctor. It took me a while to pluck up the courage to ask the doctor for this, as I felt very inferior, and as he was so busy, I didn't want to be a nuisance. I went to the physiotherapist only to be told that it was too late for me to join the present block of classes, as they were just about to finish.

Feeling unlucky and disappointed, I went to my local council-run library to get some books on childbirth. There was only one, written by a physiotherapist. Back in 1975, I rarely heard the subject of childbirth discussed. Maybe women discussed it amongst themselves, but growing up, I rarely heard the word mentioned. The book I found at the library was focused on exercise, but there was one paragraph that said you must relax during labour and to forget about modesty. There were no diagrams or pictures of a pregnant woman or her baby, only a slim woman in leotard and tights doing exercises, so this was all the information I had.

Although my mother had given birth four times, she didn't tell me much about childbirth. When I asked her, she said she couldn't remember a lot, but she did tell me that my birth at a small, private nursing home in Brisbane, Queensland, in 1948 was easy. She said she had been in the home for some hours before I was born, and the only thing that upset her was that the doctor, who lived next door, never arrived. It was left to the nurse or midwife to manage things, but my mother said I came out by myself and it wasn't painful.

When having her 4th and last child in a different private hospital, she was also upset, because the doctor said she wasn't pushing hard enough and just as the baby was being born, he knocked her out with anaesthetic. I can still remember when I was around 10 years of age going to visit her at the hospital and how unhappy she looked.

However, there is one thing that she taught my sisters and I, and this was whenever we had a period, to mark the date on the calendar, which hung in the kitchen. This became a habit all through my life and I always kept a record. When I became pregnant, eventually five times, there was never any doubt about my due dates. Having a scan was not a routine procedure back then, and it might seem strange, but I have never had one scan during five pregnancies.

About four months into my first pregnancy, I left work in a solicitor's office and stayed at home preparing for the baby. In those days, around 1975, many women still sewed their own clothes and I made my summer nighties and brunch coats (lightweight dressing gowns), for hospital, and most of the baby's clothes. I made matinee jackets and bunny rugs for the baby, both for warm weather and cooler weather. I would be in hospital for six days, which was pretty normal at that time.

Everything was ready when the time came. I had three-dozen, (36), towelling nappies, which I had washed, because I don't think many people used disposable nappies, I had never even seen one. All the baby's things were so soft and smelt really beautiful. We had a room all set up and I would go in there and open the cupboard just to delight in looking at the beautiful, little, baby clothes and all the things I had made or bought.

As my due date came closer, I packed a suitcase and I had bought myself a lovely, beauty case for toiletries to take to hospital. It was cream with gold locks and a purple, satin lining. Little did I know when I bought it, that I would use it three more times at the births of my other children. But the fifth time, I didn't need it because I stayed at home. However, as they say, that's another story.

To tell you a little about myself, I went to several, different Government-run State Schools in Brisbane, Queensland, Australia and after Grade 8 at the age of 13 years I went to a State High School for secondary education. This was in the early 1960's when life was very different. At High School, I did a commercial course concentrating on shorthand, typing and bookkeeping and after two years at High School, aged 15, I was employed for some years as a legal stenographer in a solicitor's office doing shorthand, typing and accounts.

Since the age of eight years, I had learned classical ballet and in 1966 I passed two major examinations. In 1967, I sailed to England and spent over three years dancing professionally. In between shows, I did temporary work as a legal stenographer for solicitors and barristers and various other types of businesses in London and elsewhere. In those days, if you were Australian, you had no trouble finding work in the UK.

At High School we did do a course of mothercraft lessons, when once a week, a nurse came to the school to teach us. She wore a white, nurse's uniform and veil and showed us how to bath a doll. She was very jolly, and we learned about feeding, potty training, baby clothing and hygiene. I really don't think the word "childbirth" was ever mentioned. We all had to take an exam in mothercraft and make our own book with all the leaflets she had given us.

At the time of my first pregnancy, I was very fit and still athletic from all the years of ballet training and dancing. About 2:00pm one afternoon in 1975, when I was two days past my due date, I discovered I'd had a small show of blood. I rang the doctor's surgery, and the receptionist told me he wasn't there; he was up at the hospital. So, I rang the hospital and a nursing sister said, that as this was my first baby, I didn't need to come up until about 5:00pm.

My husband was at work, so I rang and told him what was happening. I went to the toilet, my bowels moved and I had a shower. Walking around, I began to feel the strong, recurring tightening of my stomach, which I vaguely knew was called a contraction. Remembering what it said in the one article I had read, that I must relax, this is what I kept on doing. As the contraction came, I relaxed.

## Chapter One — Painful Ignorance Sets Off a Learning Curve

About 4:00pm my mother-in-law, arrived and stayed with me and I started to write down the times when the contractions started and how long they lasted. She was watching me and told me I couldn't possibly be correct as they were too close together. I wasn't at all worried and I had no fear whatsoever, I could feel the pressure inside me, and the strong pains. In actual fact, I was so relaxed I was enjoying the rhythm of the contractions because I knew the baby would soon be here. I kept on relaxing, noticing the tightening and unafraid of the sensations of birth, writing my record.

Arriving at the maternity hospital just after 5:00pm, my husband and I went inside and up to the reception counter. There was a nursing sister there, she was middle-aged, a solidly built woman, very red faced and with a red rose. She was unfriendly and spoke abruptly and told us that we would have to sit down in the waiting room as all the staff were having their dinner break.

We sat down in the waiting room and we waited for an hour. The contractions were still coming very regularly and were strong, but I managed to keep up the relaxing. After the hour was up, I could see several staff walking around behind the counter and we started to get a bit worried they had forgotten about us, because nobody acknowledged us at all. As the pains were getting stronger all the time, I went up to the desk and was told they could take me in now. I had to leave my suitcase, but could take my beauty case in with me.

Now, remembering this was 1975, you will probably think it incredible, but at this hospital, a teaching hospital, husbands were not allowed to be present in the Labour Ward for the birth of their child. Only when the midwives told them, were they allowed to come in and sit with their wives, but were sent out for any internal examinations and the birth.

The reasons given to us were that there were no male toilets in the maternity hospital. Also, if the husband fainted, the nurses couldn't be expected to have to look after him as well. We never questioned any of this. In any case, at that time, some husbands may have preferred not to be there because it just wasn't the done thing.

The door to the Labour Ward was very heavy and had a big, clear, glass panel through which you could see a corridor and doorways. The sister took me into a room on my left. She motioned for me to climb up onto a bed and she walked out. The bed was really high, and fairly narrow. There was a set of steps beside the bed, and although I am 5ft 4ins (163 centimetres) I needed to use the steps to get up on the bed. It was quite a large room and before long, two other sisters came in.

There certainly wasn't much in the way of public relations back then, as not one of these women ever introduced themselves. The youngest one told me it was her very first night as a student midwife; she didn't wear a sister's veil, but a see-through, fancy cap, like a butterfly. The other one was much older, she wore a sister's veil, but she never spoke. I had the feeling that she was learning and she seemed very hesitant in her manner and lacking confidence.

These women were not friendly either, they both stood at the bottom of the bed on which I was lying on my back. They didn't say anything, just looked at me, and the sister from the reception desk came marching into the room, it was obvious to me that she was in charge. I watched her as she marched around behind them. Coming to my left side, and without saying anything, she pulled up my top and put her hand onto my tummy and started feeling around.

"Bladder up to her eyeballs," she said.

My doctor suddenly appeared standing in the doorway on my right, but he didn't come into the room. Apparently, he'd been at another birth. He never looked at or even acknowledged me. He was watching the midwives. From where he was standing in the doorway, he addressed the sister who had her hand on my stomach. She now had her hand flat on my stomach and was moving it very quickly, sideways back and forth, in a vibrating type of movement.

## Chapter One — Painful Ignorance Sets Off a Learning Curve

Watching him, I could see he wasn't very impressed and he said to her, "What are you doing?"

"Putting froth on her wee," she answered.

Confused by this exchange, and having to look from one to the other, I didn't understand what was happening, but still the doctor never once looked at me. Finally, he gave this midwife a glaring look, and without saying another word to anybody, he turned abruptly on his heel and left the doorway leaving me wondering what this was all about.

The older midwife and the younger one left the room, and the one in charge from reception told me to get up and use the toilet, which was in the same room. As I hadn't spoken a word until now, I thought I'd try to initiate some friendly conversation with her, 'break the ice' or something like that, after all, I didn't know her from a bar of soap.

"I used to be a dancer," I said.

"Oh! Well then," she replied, "You'll have nice, tight muscles, won't you?" and she left the room.

Taken aback by this statement, I had thought the fact that I was fit was a good thing, but from what this midwife said, it sounded to me as though it could be a problem. Feeling a little deflated and uneasy, I climbed down off the bed and went to the toilet. It was a huge relief to pass urine and I really liked sitting on the toilet because as the contractions came, I felt somehow supported and I stayed in there for quite a while. I was remembering to relax as each contraction started and ran its course. The midwives had to come and knock on the toilet door and tell me to come out. *(In Chapter 3, I look at this misconception that a fit woman, necessarily has 'tight' muscles.)*

The hesitant midwife and the student wanted to examine me internally. They told me to take off all my clothes and they gave me a very short, old, grey, hospital jacket to wear. It only came to my waist and opened at the back. It had ties to hold it together. The shoulders were also open but did up with buttons. The problem was that many buttons were missing and I had a lot of trouble keeping it on.

I remembered to relax my body as the older woman, examined me internally.

In shock, she gasped and drew back in horror exclaiming, "God kid! You're almost there, you're eight centimeters."

She looked at me as though she couldn't believe it, maybe because I was so calm and relaxed. She was very flustered and said, "I can't go and ring the doctor now; he's just left, he'll think I'm drunk." They both walked out.

I really didn't understand this, I didn't have enough education, but I wasn't scared or frightened at this stage. However, none of them ever spoke to me or shared anything with me, they spoke to each other, over me, as though I wasn't there, and I, in my ignorance never asked them anything. Anyway, the impression I got was that they knew everything and they were in charge, and as a person, somehow, I was not important in any of this, it was their job.

Next to come in was the young midwifery student, she brought in quite a bit of equipment, rubber tubes and jugs. She said she had to give me an enema. Somehow, I plucked up the courage and said, "I moved my bowels before I came here." But she told me that I still had to have an enema. Also, I wouldn't be allowed to pass it on the toilet, I would have to sit on a bedpan up on the bed, as I was too far-gone.

While I was lying on my left side, she poured soapy water out of a jug, through a funnel and hose, and in through my rectum. I thought I would explode, and I did. After all the water was inside me, I had to sit up on a really high, and hard, stainless-steel bedpan to pass it. I had great difficulty maneuvering myself around the narrow, high bed and keeping my balance as I perched and squatted up on the bedpan, not an easy task at nine months pregnant, and in labour, and probably now would be considered

## Chapter One — Painful Ignorance Sets Off a Learning Curve

dangerous. Just as well my legs were very strong and I was flexible

As there was absolutely nothing to hang on to, all I could do to steady myself was to reach down with my fingertips and touch the bed for balance. I squatted up on the pan, which seemed so small, and my baby tummy seemed so big. I was hoping that I didn't make a mess, as all that water spurted out of me.

The student midwife was standing back watching me as I experienced a huge contraction, my stomach rose up and was hard as a rock and I was forced to let my head and my body fall to one side, my left, so I could fully support myself by putting my left hand flat down on the bed. With great difficulty, I was also trying to hold on to the hospital coat, constantly pulling it up onto my shoulders.

The whole time, this student midwife stood looking at me, at a distance, terrified, saying nothing, and I was very embarrassed. She never once came forward or offered any support whatsoever. As it was her first night on duty as a midwife, I could tell she was really quite frightened of me and everything else that was going on.

As the pain of another contraction reached its height, I groaned, as passing all this water was so incredibly uncomfortable. The young midwife said to me, "You won't bear down, will you?"

I raised my head and looked over at her, "No," was all I could manage to say.

Never before, in my life, had I been in an embarrassing situation like this, something you usually do in private.

She said to me, "You'll have to get off that now."

"But it isn't finished," I protested because the water was still spurting out of me into the pan.

"It doesn't matter," she said and she took away the bedpan.

As I lay down on the bed on my left side, the water kept coming out and she had to get towels and keep cleaning up. What a mess, I felt dreadfully embarrassed. Finally, it stopped and after more cleaning up, she walked out the door. I think I had a shower then, but it wasn't long after that another student midwife in a cap came in and told me she had to shave off all my pubic hair, right the way through my legs.

This was a terrible shock to me, as I didn't know anything about this procedure or why it was being done. My skin is white and fair, but my hair, at that time, was black and thick and during this whole, shaving ordeal, not once did this midwife speak to me, and by now I was really feeling like a second-class citizen.

This midwife was very rough and I was so frightened she would cut me as she dragged the razor down over my genitals. It was a stainless steel, safety razor with razor blades, like men used for shaving at that time. I had to tell her that I would hold back the folds of skin myself, so I could shield myself with my hand. I could tell she found the whole thing disgusting and distasteful, and so did I, absolutely disgusting and perverse.

In those days, women didn't wax or shave their entire pubic area like many do today. I had always needed to keep my bikini line tidy because of high cut leotards or costumes. But this was a whole new experience for me and I will never forget the abject humiliation, fear and discomfort that I felt. This particular midwife who shaved me left the room and I never saw her again, something for which I was very grateful.

Another unknown midwife came into the room, and told me that I had to move to another room across the corridor. The short, hospital jacket was still very annoying and falling off my shoulders, and it only just reached to my navel. She saw the difficulty I was having keeping it on, but never once offered to help me. I also never dared ask for a better jacket, this wasn't in my make up at that time.

After climbing down from the bed, I was standing there, naked from the waist down. As I had to walk across the corridor, I knew people might see me through the glass door that led from this Labour Ward out into the waiting room. I asked this midwife for something to put around me, but I could see she was impatient

## Chapter One — Painful Ignorance Sets Off a Learning Curve

for me to get going. However, she could also see I wasn't going to budge and very reluctantly she found a clean sheet that I unfolded and wrapped around my waist, I picked up my beauty case, managing to hold onto the jacket and the sheet and followed her.

What an enormous shock I had when I walked through the doorway into this other large room opposite. There were renovations going on, it was a building site, with large sheets of clear plastic hanging down from the ceiling to the floor. As I came in, I actually saw the face of a workman; he gave me a strange sort of smile and quickly ducked back under what seemed like a canvas wall. I was very glad I had the sheet around me. I could hardly even make out where this midwife was leading me. As I looked down, I saw the concrete floor had been dug up, it was all rubble, but a pathway had been left in the middle with cracked pieces of concrete, dirt and rubble bordering either side.

Following the midwife, picking my way along, finally, by a circuitous route we arrived at the centre of this room and another high bed. There was a lot of equipment in this room, much of it covered in plastic sheeting. The midwife left and I sat on the bed looking around me, there was a big clock on the wall in front and I could see large lights on tall stands and stainless-steel trolleys and equipment. It was a stark and cold room and there was nothing to look at except the clock. It was like an operating theatre.

The younger student midwife came in, and suddenly, without saying anything to me, she roughly shoved a horn hard into the side of my stomach. I gasped in pain, as this really hurt; she said she was listening to the baby's heartbeat. It was after 7:00pm and soon my husband came into the room. It was the first time I'd seen him, he'd been in the waiting room all the time, but he hadn't had anything to eat, so he left to go home and get some dinner.

The bed was very hard, more like a table, and I only had one, very flat pillow. I remained there alone with the contractions coming regularly. My husband came back about 8:00pm and I was lying on my side. I was feeling well and continuing with the relaxing. Sometime later, the doctor came into the room with the first sister

I had seen in the reception area.

He didn't speak to my husband or I, but he felt my tummy and said to the sister, "It can come down more yet," and he left.

That was all, he hardly acknowledged us, and I felt it was as though somehow, we weren't worth talking to. The sister followed him out, but she turned back at the doorway and said to my husband, "She won't be smiling soon."

It was nearly 10:00pm and the pain was much stronger. A midwife came in, I hadn't seen her before, but she had a pretty face.

She quickly put an injection into my leg, "What was that?" I asked her.

"It's pethidine, for the pain," she answered, "if you don't have it now, you can't have it later."

Before long, I was finding it hard to keep my eyes open. Fighting to hold my head up, as the contractions came, I found I couldn't relax as my body was falling all over the place. My husband sat beside me and I could sense his concern, as it was very abnormal for me to be like this.

The sister from reception and the older one came into the room and they told my husband to leave. They instructed me to lie flat on my back, draw up my knees and let my legs fall out, as they had to give me another internal examination. But I could see them doing something else to me. Suddenly, I heard water spurt out of me and the sisters were laughing.

Managing to prop myself up on my elbows, I said, "What are you doing?" The sister from reception said to me, "You just about gave her a bath." They went out laughing and I was alone. The pain now became overpowering, and as a contraction came, I didn't know how I could bear it, I didn't know what to do. I didn't know where my husband was; he hadn't come back in after they went out. There was nobody there for me to ask.

In my mind, I was crying out, 'Where is the doctor, when will he come?'

## Chapter One — Painful Ignorance Sets Off a Learning Curve

I couldn't understand why he wasn't here with me. I was fighting to stay awake, and the pain was now excruciating. I wondered if it would ever end.

At one stage, the sister from reception came and stood in the doorway. She looked as though she was in a big hurry.

I said to her, "When will the doctor come?" She said, "When I call him," and she just went away.

Suddenly, there was a commotion in another room; a woman was crying out and the midwives were shouting at her, "There's no use crying, that's not going to do you any good." I thought another woman must have been having a baby. The awful noise went on for quite a while. I wondered if the same thing was in store for me.

Around 11:00pm the pretty midwife who gave me the pethidine and a new sister came into the room. I realised the shift must have changed. The new sister had black hair sticking out from under her veil. She was limping, and I saw her big toe sticking up, all bandaged. She had a rubber thong, (sandal), on that foot and a lace-up brown shoe on the other.

They wanted me to get onto my back, I was in agony, and as I rolled over, the pretty one looked at my stomach. As I was having a contraction, it was hard and tight. She said to the other one, "Funny shape." This frightened me, and I said, "Is something wrong?" But neither of them answered me and they walked out the door. Now I was alone and fear started to engulf me. I kept thinking, 'How could anyone relax with this pain?'

Sometime later, the pretty one and the one with the thong on her foot, came marching back in and told me that now I was going to push. They were so bossy and they roughly pushed my legs up towards my shoulders and told me to grip my knees. Because of my big tummy, I could hardly reach my knees. They instructed me to take a deep breath and hold it, put my chin on my chest and push down into my bottom.

"Push, push," they shouted.

"Come on, you're not pushing hard enough." "Push, push."

"No, you're pushing in your throat, that's no good." "Come on, get really mad with your baby; push him out."

"Push, push."

"Push, push, don't waste a contraction, push, push."

"Push down hard in your bottom like you want to go to the toilet." "Push down, push down, push down hard."

The pain and pressure around my vagina were unbearable, and from gripping my knees in that position, and with my chin down on my chest, I think it had cut off my oxygen and I could hardly get my breath. Exhausted and frightened, I thought I was going to die. I'd pushed as hard as I could, but nothing was happening.

Pushing into my rectum confused me and I wondered how on earth the baby would get out as that part of me was practically flat on the bed. Also, what if I pushed the baby out and the doctor wasn't there? This was another thought torturing my mind adding to my stress. They let me lie down.

"When will the doctor come?" I asked the untidy one.

"When I call him," she said and they both walked out the door. I felt as though I couldn't do anything right.

Fear and dread now invaded my whole body, which became stiff as a board, leaving me petrified and afraid to move. Imagining the worst, I was sure that my baby and I would die. The contractions still kept coming, the pain convulsing my body as my back arched and my head was thrown back because of the tension and the strength of the contraction. There was no way I could relax, as I was now full of terror. My body seemed paralysed, cold and stiff. But they came in again. Once more I had to grip my knees and push.

"Push down hard."

"Push down in your bottom like you want to go to the toilet." "Come on, push down hard," and again, "push down."

## Chapter One — Painful Ignorance Sets Off a Learning Curve

While I was pushing and gripping my knees, I saw the doctor come into the room and they let me lie down. He didn't speak to me, but I watched as he moved things around. He noticed the sister with the thong on her foot and said something to her and she laughed. Other midwives had come into the room and they were all walking towards the wall opposite, well away from where I was lying.

They were talking together when suddenly the one with the sore toe walked towards me and without any warning, in one dramatic movement, she did something and half the bed disappeared. Shocked, frightened and confused, I had no idea what was happening. Quickly, I had to scramble backwards as I was now sitting only on a small ledge, the top part of the bed. My genitals and my tummy felt like they were hanging over space and I could see the floor beneath. I was speechless and terrified.

Walking towards me, she was holding a pole and she put it into the lower left corner of what remained of the bed. The same was done on the right side. Some sort of white coverings were pulled up over my legs. The two poles had loops attached to the top of them and she took hold of my left leg, pulled it apart and put it up through the loop. The doctor took hold of my right leg, but for some reason, as he did so, my leg flew out towards him. I think it was some symptom of my fear, a reflex, because I was so tense and stiff and I didn't have any idea what was going on. From all the pushing, my eyes felt as though they were bulging out of my head. What a pathetic spectacle I must have looked.

But as my leg flew out, I think the doctor thought I meant to kick him. I hadn't done it on purpose, but I was so afraid of what was going to happen to me. He put my right leg through the loop. Now I know they are called "stirrups."

When both my legs were strung up through the loops, the doctor told me to move my bottom forward to the edge of the table. I didn't want to, it seemed like this would be the end of me. But there was no getting away, so I had to surrender to whatever was in store for me. I was in a pitiful position, lost, alone, and at this point, I abandoned all hope. I couldn't speak because I was so afraid and knew that I was about to die.

Now all the sisters were in the room, standing in a group opposite me and talking to each other. They were leaning against the back wall under the clock. Nobody was with me, not one of them was with me and not one of them spoke to me. At some time, the doctor put a catheter in me, because I heard water draining out into a bucket and I also saw him hold up a big needle to inject me.

Suddenly, the sister with the thong on her foot came rushing forward, "Push, push down hard," she yelled at me really loudly, "Now push down hard."

With my legs strung up, I pushed again with all my might, as hard as I could. The doctor said nothing, he was sitting on a stool between my legs, but he turned and glared after her as though she'd lost her mind. She limped back to the group standing against the wall.

There was the sound of scissors cutting, followed by the agony of a terrible pressure inside me, high up inside me, first pushing hard, deep inside me, then pulling back, tearing, twisting and turning. I'd never felt any pain like it, but I had told myself that no matter what, I wouldn't make a noise. No matter what they did to me, even though I died, I would not give them the satisfaction of hearing me cry out.

Where this thought came from, I couldn't say, but I felt nobody had helped me or cared less about me, neither the midwives nor the doctor. So, throughout the whole ordeal, I never made a sound. The whole experience was so macabre and never in my wildest dreams would I have thought that this type of thing could be done to a woman having a baby.

The pain stopped, but I heard nothing, no cry, so I knew the baby must be dead. I knew that it couldn't have survived that violence. Struggling, I managed to prop myself up on my elbows so I could see what the doctor was doing. He had my baby in his hands and was bending over, but I couldn't see the baby's face.

## Chapter One — Painful Ignorance Sets Off a Learning Curve

There was a cry, and the untidy sister came forward to take it away. The doctor told me it was a boy, but I never had the chance to see it. These were the only words he ever said to me. It was some time before midnight.

He sat between my legs, which were still strung up, and he started stitching me. The sisters had all left the room. It was terribly painful and I could see the bloodied scissors as every now and again, he placed them into a pocket on the covering that was on my leg. The pain was so excruciating and, in the silence, my head, which was flat on the bed started to move of its own accord from one side to the other. Strange, I knew it was happening and I tried to stop it, but I couldn't.

Despite my not wanting to make a noise, every now and then I heard myself moan because the place where he was continually stitching was so sensitive. It seemed to take a long time, but finally he stood up and left the room. My legs were still attached to the poles, and after he left, my head stopped moving and I wondered if I could take my legs down myself as I couldn't feel them.

It was some time before the pretty midwife came in, but I soon realised she was a very cold and unfeeling person. She'd somehow replaced the lower end of the bed, as she took down my legs, removed the white coverings and crossed one of my legs over the other. Feeling very stiff, cold, thirsty and hungry I was still too frightened to move. The baby was brought in and put into a small cot beside me. My husband came in and we looked at our baby. Hardly believing this little stranger was mine, I ran my finger gently down his cheek. He was a beautiful, little boy and his eyes were wide open and he was alert, looking around. The midwife told me that I wouldn't be allowed to hold him for two days, as he had to be cot rested. He weighed 8lbs 2oz (3.6 kilos).

My husband left and once again I caressed my baby's cheek, as we were alone. They took him away again, and the pretty, cold, nurse gave me a wash. I wish she hadn't bothered, because the water in the bowl was cold, and despite my saying I had my own face washer in my beauty case, she used the rough, calico covering off a vomit bowl, which had been sitting on a locker beside the bed.

It wasn't hard to see she was sour at having to wash me. She dried me very quickly and sprinkled me with baby powder, which all caked on my damp skin. I put on my own clean nightie and somehow, I climbed off the bed and onto a trolley. I held back the plastic sheeting that was hanging down as, with a lot of difficulty, she wheeled the trolley out of the room and down the corridor into the ward.

As I was a private patient, I was in a two-bed room and I climbed slowly into the bed. I was feeling very hungry, but intimidated as I was, wouldn't have dared ask for anything to eat. I'd had nothing to eat or drink for at least 12 hours.

It was dark in the room, but there was a jug of water on the bedside table. I reached up to pour some out into a glass. But the lid hadn't been put on properly and it fell into the glass, water splashing all over the bed and me, but I really didn't care. I might have slept a little, but I was in a lot of pain and too frightened to even change position. I really didn't know what had happened and could hardly believe I'd had a baby. I felt very lonely the rest of that night.

About 5:00am a lady came in with a tea trolley and gave me a cup of tea. I had never tasted anything so wonderful in all my life; it was one cup of tea that I have never forgotten. Only, there was a problem, the bed and the back of my nightie from the hem to the neck, were soaked with blood. I hadn't even noticed it because I'd been too scared to move all night. The tea lady called a nurse, who was a nurse's aide. She kindly helped me to sit in a chair, took the sheet off the bed and, very concerned, carried it away. Shortly afterwards, she came back accompanied by a sister.

Unfortunately, it was the untidy sister who had been there at the birth; only today she had on both brown, lace up shoes. I found it difficult to sit down and drink my wonderful tea, because I was so sore and stiff, therefore I stood up. She looked at me and told me that I could go and have a shower.

## Chapter One — Painful Ignorance Sets Off a Learning Curve

So, I drank my tea, picked up my beauty case and went into the shower. It was so painful to walk and I was a little weak and dizzy, but I made it into the bathroom and washed myself all over. The shower felt marvellous, and as I came out, the untidy sister was standing in the corridor outside my room with another sister whom I hadn't seen previously. They were talking, but I could hear what they were saying, and she was being reprimanded for telling me to have a shower. I think I was supposed to be still in bed.

During the day, my parents came to see me and we were able to see my baby son. In those days, they had one central nursery and all the babies were kept in the one place. You weren't allowed to have your baby in your room, only at feed time. When visitors came, you stood outside the nursery in front of a big glass window and the nurse brought your baby for your visitors to see. People could only see your baby through the glass. They weren't allowed to touch it or handle it in any way. The sister wheeled my baby over in his little cot and for the first time I saw the words, "Kielland's forceps" written in big letters attached to one end. I didn't know what it meant, but I felt so sad for my baby all alone in there.

Later that day, a friend came to see me. She had been a midwife and explained to me all about my baby's delivery. She said he was stuck in the birth canal because he didn't rotate. He was the wrong way around. They call it a "POP" and it meant Persistent Occipito Posterior, his spine on my spine, so they had to use forceps to turn him and pull him out. At that time, I accepted everything she said.

I wanted to breast feed my baby and during the day, I noticed that my breasts were getting really big and hard. They would wheel the babies out into the ward in their little cots and put them in a straight line, bumper to bumper, down the middle of the long corridor. The mothers would come out and get their baby every four hours to feed. Only I didn't have my baby. The next day my breasts were even more painful and hard as footballs and when I came out of the shower there was a glass horn with a rubber bulb standing on my locker. I didn't even know what it was.

I asked a nurse, and she told me it was a breast pump and she showed me how to use it to express milk. I started expressing and I was filling up a glass with a lot of milk. Not knowing what to do with it, I poured it down the sink. Later that afternoon a pediatrician came to see me. He spoke kindly to me and said even though it had been a forceps delivery, my baby was perfect and that I would be able to feed him at the next feed. I was so pleased and happy I could hardly wait. But when the babies were wheeled down the hallway, mine wasn't there.

Going down to the nursery, I tried to get the attention of the sister who was inside with the babies. She seemed very stressed, but opened the door and listened to what I said. She went away and came back with another sister who told me in no uncertain terms that on no account could I have my baby yet.

My heart sank, because I was so disappointed. I said to her that the pediatrician had been and told me that I could feed my baby that afternoon at the next feed. She said that obviously he didn't know the rules of this hospital. I was very confused as I thought his instructions would somehow take precedence and I became very upset.

I broke down and started to cry. They just walked away, went into the nursery and left me there. I sank down onto a seat outside the glass window of the nursery and couldn't stop crying. I was trying to see where my baby was, and which one he was, as I had hardly seen him since he was born. The first nurse saw me and must have taken pity. She wheeled my baby out to me and said I could give him his bottle, I think it was sugar and water, but he had to stay lying down in the cot, I couldn't pick him up. Feeding him, I touched his little hands and arms and he drank well.

It had been difficult holding in my disappointment and my pain, but that night, when the lights were out, I put my face into the pillow and just cried uncontrollably, I couldn't help it. The pediatrician and the tea lady were the only people who spoke to me as though I was a human being.

## Chapter One — Painful Ignorance Sets Off a Learning Curve

The next morning at feed time, my baby was brought to me. But it was the sister from reception who brought him in. This woman was very intimidating and I had a strong feeling of resentment deep within me because she was possessively holding my baby and I, as his mother, hadn't even held him yet. She was going to show me how to breast-feed and she said because my nipples were so small, I would have to use the "twin" position.

She put the baby on his back, on a pillow and pushed this under my armpit, so his head was under my breast. I had to lean forward and push my nipple into his mouth. As she roughly pinched and squeezed my nipple, she said, "You've got nothing, you have to make something."

Needless to say, this didn't help any confidence I might have had. As my nipple touched his lips, he immediately opened his mouth, but he couldn't seem to latch on. My breasts were very hard and painful. After he fed from one side, I had to put the pillow under my other arm, lie him down on his back and repeat the process on the other side.

At his subsequent feeds I persevered with this positioning. I had to sit on the bed and lean forward all the time and this really put pressure on all my stitches. It wasn't a comfortable position for me to feed the baby, so the next day I started off in this position, but decided to do what came naturally, I sat on a pillow on the chair next to my bed, put a pillow on my lap and simply cradled my baby in my arm and he took the breast very easily, small nipple and all.

It seems ridiculous and strict, but you were only allowed to breast feed for 10 minutes each side, and the time was just about up, but because I had been changing my positioning, he hadn't really had enough time sucking. We were just settling down when a sister came in and demanded I give up my baby as the time was up and she had to get the babies back to the nursery.

I protested and said to her that I hadn't really had enough time to feed him, but she was adamant she had to test weigh him and to this day, I will never forget how he cried and his little face screwed up in frustration and disappointment as she took him from my breast. She literally had to pull my nipple out of his mouth, and I saw his frantic look and the milk that was there. I heard him crying loudly all the way down the corridor as she took him away, I think this was because he had finally been happy and getting some milk, warmth and comfort.

Strangely, of all the pain I had endured, this was the worst. Even though I had travelled, earned my own money and lived overseas independently, I was totally unprepared for this situation. I had no coping skills, I had no words, no defence, nobody to help me or give me advice, I felt so sad and helpless and knew I had been judged by these people as an inadequate mother. But it was the callousness and cruelty of the place, and yet I had to somehow find the strength, hide my true feelings and stay there while these people were in charge of me.

This midwife brought my baby back to me and told me that the test weigh showed he'd had nothing. She gave me a bottle with milk in it and told me to feed it to him. I was so confused, still expressing plenty of breast milk, but unable to feed him and now my nipples were very sore.

I stayed in the hospital for six days, which was then pretty normal. Once when I started to feed my baby, he dirtied his nappy and it all ran out. I carried him back to the central nursery and asked the nurse if she could change him. I'll never forget how rough she was with him and how angry I felt as I watched her; because I could easily have changed his nappy myself if I'd had access to some. I was at least capable of doing that. She told me that if he did it again, I was to keep feeding him and not to bring him back.

Apart from the need to have access to my baby to breast feed him properly, this incident was to be the catalyst the following year, after the birth of my second child, for my writing to the hospital and requesting that they introduce rooming in, which means you can care for your own baby in the ward.

## Chapter One — Painful Ignorance Sets Off a Learning Curve

There were other women in the area wanting the same thing, to have access to their babies. Despite many arguments for and against, I think it was introduced about two years later and now it is common practice. But I know of one doctor who was on the hospital board and he angrily said to me, "You'll never see rooming in at this hospital."

On my last day in the hospital a sister came down and gave me a lecture about breast feeding and topping up with the bottle, because while my nipples were so sore, this is what I had been doing. She was an old grouch and told me that I had to do one or the other, that she'd tried to do both herself and it didn't work. All I wanted to do was get out of there and go home. Finally, it was time to leave and I was so pleased when I saw my husband in the waiting room and I went to the nursery and asked for my baby as I was going home.

I wheeled my baby in his cot up to my room, took off all his hospital clothes and for the first time, I looked at him properly, he was now mine. I put on his new clothes, wrapped him in a rug and walked out to my husband in the waiting room. Nobody was around so we just left and I didn't say goodbye to anyone. My husband was very relieved to see us and when we were in the car park, after six days, he had his very first nurse of his son.

I settled in at home, but I was still dealing with very sore nipples and my bowels hadn't moved the entire time I'd been in the hospital. The day before I left a sister gave me a whole bottle of white medicine to take with me, and I'd tried suppositories, but still nothing happened.

The second day at home, my husband and I decided I needed an enema. He borrowed the equipment from his mother and we managed to get me moving again. I took my baby to the Maternal and Child Welfare to have him weighed and he was putting on weight very well.

But I lacked confidence in breast-feeding because I couldn't tell if he'd had enough breast milk and I was frightened he wasn't getting adequate nourishment. It was just inexperience as I know now that both of us were doing fine, and despite being told that all was well, my confidence as a mother was zero, and I decided to put my baby on the bottle at around six weeks.

It was such a relief to be back in my clean and comfortable home and to have peace and quiet. After this first birth experience, there was something that I wanted to know as a matter of interest and I asked my friend, who had been a midwife at that hospital, about some of the sisters who were there at my son's birth. She knew all of them, and when I asked her if any of them had children, she told me that not one was a mother.

There may have been midwives at that hospital, who were kind, but I started to think, it is an unknown. You don't know who will be on duty or whom you will get when you go into labour, and as the doctor is hardly ever there during that time, you are just alone.

Thankfully, the situation is different these days with husbands or partners and other support persons allowed to be with the mother during labour and birth. But at the time I first gave birth, that was not the situation and husbands or partners or other family members were not allowed to be present at this hospital.

*Chapter Two*

# A LITTLE LEARNING WENT A LONG WAY

My husband and I wanted a family, so the following year in 1976 I was again pregnant and because I had accepted everything that happened to me with the birth of my first child, and the fact that he didn't rotate, I went again to the same obstetrician and the same local hospital. We knew of no alternative. Attending the Physiotherapy Classes was a top priority for me this time and I asked the doctor for a referral. He wrote it out for me and said, "It doesn't seem to make any difference." I wasn't put off by this remark and so I enrolled in the Physiotherapy Classes.

The Physiotherapist was a very motherly woman who'd had six children. She taught the class, expectant mothers and husbands or partners, about muscles and contractions and we learned how to recognise a relaxed muscle and a tense muscle. We'd tighten the muscles in our arms and feel that sensation and then we'd relax them and feel the difference. Quite a lot of the time she would refer to a Dr Grantly Dick-Read. She'd say, Grantly Dick-Read said this, and Dr Grantly Dick-Read said that.

With regard to breathing, as the contractions peaked, we could pant softly through our mouths, as this helped to stop you from holding your breath because of the pain. Otherwise, it was just to breathe normally and relax all your muscles as you exhaled. If you breathed this way, you knew that the baby was getting enough oxygen through the cord. She also told us about how the cervix became gradually thinner closer to the birth (effacement) and when contractions started it would dilate (become wider), eventually to 10 centimeters. *(About the size of a small melon. There are many illustrations you can now find on the internet about effacement and cervical dilation).*

Whilst I appreciated her teaching, I thought she painted a very rosy picture of hospital childbirth. All the participants were first time mothers, except me. Sometimes I couldn't help myself and I said something like, "I didn't find that." She said to me that if I wanted to say something, just to let her know and she'd speak to me after the class, but on my own. I realised she didn't want me to frighten anyone.

I honestly don't know the answer to this dilemma and it has been the same for me with this book I have written. You want to warn people to be aware, but you don't want to make them afraid, because not everyone will meet the same staff or the same circumstances.

Sometimes after the class this physiotherapist would speak with me and I'd told her a bit about my first birth experience. I told her that I thought some of the midwives weren't very empathetic and it shocked me when she said, "Then they shouldn't be there." She told me I'd had a "raw" experience.

At my very last antenatal visit with the obstetrician, and because I was dreading going through all the pain again, I asked him if this coming birth would be the same as the last. I could tell I'd caught him by surprise, because he looked completely blank. I don't think he even remembered my first birth at all. Quickly, he started to turn back through the pages of my file and he muttered something unintelligible. I let it go.

One Saturday afternoon, I was in the laundry doing some washing when I started to feel a lot of pain in my back. It was about two days before my due date, and I'd had no problems during the pregnancy. I hadn't had a show of blood this time, just the pains in my back and I thought that I was probably starting labour, but I wasn't sure.

## Chapter One — Painful Ignorance Sets Off a Learning Curve

I called my husband at work, and we went up to the hospital about 2:00pm. I couldn't believe how unlucky I was when the sister at the reception was the red-faced, solid woman whom I'd known when I had my first baby. Our little boy was with us, about 14 months old now and walking well. She told us to sit down; we were the only people in the waiting room.

There was a square, wooden, coffee table in this reception area and it had an arrangement of artificial flowers sunken into the middle. My little boy was amusing himself and having fun walking around this table trying to reach the flowers in the centre. He couldn't have possibly reached them because his little arms were too short.

But this sister yelled out to us from across the reception area, "Well, will you be satisfied when he breaks them?"

We were so mortified and embarrassed and, under his breath, my husband angrily commented that there was no way our son could possibly reach the flowers. I started to think that this woman was just a very bitter, old bully. I disliked her intensely.

We didn't wait very long and she told me to come in to the Prep Room. As I was lying on the bed, I saw my doctor in the doorway. I hadn't rung the surgery this time, as it was a Saturday so I just came straight to the hospital. I said to him that I thought I might be in labour and he said, "Well, you're not getting out," and he left without another word.

I had to have the enema again, but this time I could use the toilet. I'd also cut off a lot of my pubic hair with scissors, so the shave wasn't so bad. A very nice sister with a white veil came into the room accompanied by another midwife. She explained that she was going to give me a vaginal examination. This was quite gentle, but she was having trouble feeling my cervix.

The sister from reception came into the room and stood on my left. She seemed to be senior to the other one and she kept saying impatiently, "Go on, go on." I could see the nice sister's face, and I could see she didn't like this. I was lying flat on my back; my legs were pulled up and opened out.

The sister from reception put her left hand down low, under my baby, and her other one right up the top, under my breasts. I didn't know what she was doing, but without any warning, she suddenly pressed down hard on me with all her weight and at the same time, violently moved my unborn baby up and down. She kept telling the other one what to do.

It was so sudden and I was so frightened and couldn't breathe from the intense pressure on my stomach, and I cried out. Again, she did the same thing and I could hear the water inside me sloshing and squelching as she pressed heavily down on me. I cried out as I gasped for air. Did she do this to facilitate the examination or did she try to break my water?

I've asked other midwives, but they don't know. It may just have been one of this woman's own "special" procedures, not something they are taught. Later on, I complained about this to the hospital board, because it was so violent and I felt it could have damaged or dislodged the placenta, it was so rough. They did acknowledge my letter, which mentioned other issues, but never addressed this incident.

Even though I had only been a legal secretary, I would think of this as an assault, because somehow through my experiences, I was becoming more aware and less naïve about what was being done to my body. I think at that time they thought they could do anything to you because there really was nobody there on your side to witness anything thus leaving the mother very vulnerable.

The sister from reception told me that I wasn't ready yet and would have to go back into the maternity ward, as I was only three centimetres dilated. I decided that I would keep walking up and down the corridor as I felt this would be good for me. My husband took our son home to his grandparents.

I walked up and down the ward until about 6:00pm when I felt warm blood coming from my vagina. I looked and I had lost the mucus plug, so I told a nurse and was taken into the labour ward.

The contractions were quite strong, but I had been putting into practice all that I'd learned from the classes and I'd been relaxing with them all afternoon. I think too that keeping upright helped me even though I was still overcoming the shock of what that sister had done to me.

In the labour ward, I was in a different room this time, it was smaller and I didn't want to lie flat on my back. There was only one pillow so I asked a nurse if I could have another one so I could sit more upright. She told me she would get one from the other room, but if another mother came in, I would have to give it up. Thankfully, I was the only mother in the entire labour ward that night.

My husband returned and was sitting with me and a midwife had come in and was talking with us. This was a new experience, but all she could talk about was her bad back and her constant pain. My husband, wasn't impressed at all, and after she had left, he said under his breath, "She shouldn't even be here."

A short while later, this midwife wanted to examine me. My husband was sent out and after the examination, she said I was six centimetres dilated. I think she rang my doctor to inform him as I could hear her speaking on the phone outside. Coming back into the room she told me that while my membranes were intact, I wouldn't do anything, so she was going to rupture them.

The baby lies in an amniotic sack that is full of water. This helps to protect the baby, but only in two of my births have the membranes been able to rupture of their own accord. Hospitals seem to want to rupture the membranes because this makes things happen faster. But it is more difficult for the mother as, after the membranes are ruptured, the contractions become very severe, very suddenly. Also, there are risks with this practice.

Anyway, she told me that I could have pethidine, but I refused knowing how it made me feel at my last birth. Again, I had a lecture that if I didn't have it now, I couldn't have it later. Still, I refused and I don't think she liked it.

I can't say if this affected what happened next, but I didn't question her about rupturing the membranes. This never came up in the classes with the physiotherapist, so I was just submissive. This midwife also told me that my baby was POP.

I said to her, you mean "Persistent Occipito Posterior." She got a shock.

It wasn't painful when she broke my water, it was the one with the bad back, but she seemed to have her entire hand up in my vagina for a long time and without warning, she started to prod and poke me really hard and high up around my cervix. This was intensely painful and I cried out, but this didn't stop her. It was cruel, and I even put my hands down to try and protect myself and I remember saying, "Stop, please stop". If she didn't like my refusal of pethidine, she certainly wreaked her vengeance on my cervix.

Within my mind, this painful, internal procedure contributed to my now changing attitude and the chain of events that followed. I again wondered if this was a standard procedure or another assault by a midwife practising her own brand of treatment.

After she went out, I was left shaking in shock. My husband came into the room and I burst into tears and he put his arms around me as I sobbed uncontrollably. Since they broke the membranes, I was now having really strong contractions, but I relaxed with each one. I felt relieved after crying and kept telling myself to persevere this time with the relaxation. My husband rubbed my back and I found this very comforting.

We were alone in that quiet room for some time. My husband mostly sat in a chair pulled in to my right side of the bed with his head in his hands. I wasn't at all talkative; I didn't have the energy because I was dealing with the huge contractions and actively concentrating on keeping my whole body relaxed.

The contractions were now so strong I didn't know how I could go on. Once, my arms went up with a strong contraction as it reached its peak. It was as though I was trying to grab onto something, but a voice in my head kept on saying, "Come on, keep on, they say it works, you've gone this far, what have you got to lose, relax, keep on," and I lowered my arms again and relaxed them on the bed.

I was feeling so many strange sensations, but I didn't let them frighten me, I reached a stage where I knew it was relaxation or nothing, and the strange thing was that the more I did it, the more I wanted to do it and the more confident I became.

I can't say how I knew to start coaching myself, or where this came from, but relaxation with the contractions had been a technique the physiotherapist taught us and I was able to apply it. As I was coaching myself, my whole stomach suddenly started doing a somersault. I had been sitting in a semi-reclining position, supported by two pillows and I had no trouble with getting enough air. I looked down at my stomach and I saw this movement happen under the sheet.

It was corkscrew-like, smooth, sweeping and without any effort on my part. I wondered if this was the baby's head rotating, it felt like it rolled over and its head burrowed down. I simply didn't know. After that last internal examination, I had begun to think that the longer the midwives stayed away from me, the less pain I would have.

I noticed the contractions had changed. There was a lot of pressure and I wondered if this was my uterus beginning to push. It might have been sometime around 10:30pm we had heard a lot of laughing and talking. It was the shift changing. The sister with the bad back came and stood in the doorway just watching me. My husband was sitting beside the bed; his elbows were on the cover and his head still in his hands, I think he was praying.

In dealing with these different contractions, I didn't know if it was pushing or not, because I had never felt it before. I was consciously willing this sister in the doorway not to come into the room. She was the one who had hurt me so much, and I just stayed quiet. My eyes were half closed and my head was slightly bowed, but I could see her over to my left, just standing there.

She stood there for some time leaning against the wall, arms folded across her waist observing me. I was very quiet and to her, it probably looked like I was half asleep.

In my mind, I was directing my thoughts at her, 'Stay away; go away; leave me alone.'

My contractions were fierce and sometimes I felt like I would break in two from all the pressure. She never said anything to us or came into the room, and I was utterly relieved when I saw her turn and walk away.

Maybe too, in my mind I remembered how last time I had been forced to push for so long and it had been so painful. Flat on my back, with my legs tied up in the air, this was a mental picture that now filled me with terror. I wanted to keep that away for as long as I could.

I was feeling the pressure from my uterus and I could actually see my tummy rising up high and hard under the sheet and when the contraction was over I completely relaxed. There were breaks of relaxation before another contraction came. It was like, press, press, press, in one continued movement out and open, and then complete relaxation, but I was not doing it, it was my uterus. I was just going along with it when it made me press out.

The pressure built up even more and I could feel myself expanding. It was like press, press, and press out, expansion, expansion and complete rest and relaxation. This went on for quite a while. There was a rhythm.

Pressing out Pressing open

Expanding from inside

Breathing and relaxing until the next contraction. I could hear someone making loud noises in a cupboard in the corridor, which backed onto the wall of this room, and I wished they'd stop.

I thought it was after 11:00pm when my uterus pressed out very strongly. About the same time, I felt a big, wide expansion of my vagina and from being quite sleepy and limp, I felt very alert because it felt like something had completely given way. I decided I would call out to whomever was in the hallway.

"Sister, I think the baby's coming."

She was an older woman, in a veil, we hadn't even seen her before.

As she came into the room, she said, "I was just cleaning out the cupboard and coming in to check on you."

She pulled back the sheet and went into shock. "Oh! Oh!" she shouted and threw up her arms.

Turning to my husband she pointed to him and said, "You, out."

Afterwards, I would say to him how badly I felt because he had been the only one with me all along. He quickly removed himself.

Next, I think she pressed an emergency bell as it was ringing loudly all through the ward and in a few seconds about six young nurses flew in through the doorway. All in white, they reminded me of the swans in "Swan Lake". They were well trained and settled at the foot of the bed in close formation. Another younger midwife came in and stood by my left side. I was still half sitting, leaning back against the pillows.

"Don't push, don't push," the first, older one said to me. "She's not pushing," said the sister at my side.

The older one had called out for someone to ring my doctor. I really didn't know it, but the baby's head was just inside the opening of my vagina.

"Get me gloves, get me gloves," shouted the older woman. She was in a real state. "Oh!" she shouted looking at me, "and she's not even draped."

It was quite some time before I had another contraction, which was just as well. But with the next one, the baby's head just slipped through and out of my vagina. At least that's what I think happened from the look on all the nurses' faces, the ones who were at the foot of the bed. I wasn't able to see anything going on down there.

"Oh! Oh!" they exclaimed as the baby's head just slid out with no effort at all from me. I watched their faces, which were expressing a sort of rapture and awe.

There had been no force or pushing from me at all, just the pressure from my uterus. The sister at my side said to them, "See what relaxation can do."

One of them said, "I think it's the way she's sitting."

My doctor had arrived and he stood against the wall just inside the doorway. I could see him surveying the room, which seemed full of nurses.

The older sister said to him, "I've done this much, I may as well do the rest."

I thought to myself, how untrue this was, because she hadn't done anything at all.

Next thing, the sister at my side slammed down a big, black mask over my face. I was trying to see what was happening at the other end of the bed.

The older sister was saying, "Oh! Which way is it, left or right?"

I could see that she was very flustered, maybe because the doctor and all the others were watching her.

She started pulling and I started to yell, because she was hurting me.

I couldn't breathe with the sister at my side putting so much heavy pressure onto the mask on my face. I had never even seen this mask until now and never used it once. Putting my hands on the mask, I was desperate to get some air and I pushed it off. Unfortunately, it connected with her stomach and she said, "You didn't have to do that."

Now I saw the doctor walk over as the older sister was in a panic and so was I. "Relax!" the sister at my side shouted at me, the one with the mask.

### Chapter One — Painful Ignorance Sets Off a Learning Curve

"Relax!" she shouted at me again.

At that moment, the baby must have been born, because I heard my daughter cry immediately. It was some time before midnight.

I could see the doctor and the older midwife handling my baby.

He came up to me and said accusingly, "Didn't you tell anyone you wanted to push?" Not knowing how on earth to explain it at this stage, I didn't answer him.

However, it seemed I would need a few stitches.

Now that I have given birth to three more children, without any stitches, I know that the sister put too much traction on my baby before my final contraction had finished. In other words, she didn't allow for the vagina to fully expand or wait to co-ordinate the final contraction with my uterus. She took over from me, pulling too hard, and it hurt, but I didn't work this out until later.

I felt so elated, I couldn't get over it, I had done it. I was able to hold my little girl straight away. They said she was 9lbs 2ozs (4.13kilos). One of the nurses who stood at the foot of the bed came and asked me how I did it, I just said it was relaxation with the contractions.

As the older sister and the doctor walked out the door, I heard her remark, "I've never seen a baby born without a push; she had no pain."

That was also very untrue, because my uterus had pushed and called on my muscles to help, but I hadn't interfered or forced anything to happen. As for pain, I had plenty, but this woman wouldn't know because she hadn't ever been in the room until I called out. I still had a lot of learning and thinking to do, but it was so wonderful to experience a natural, spontaneous, vaginal birth.

After the birth, when everybody left, another midwife made me some toast and a cup of tea. I was very grateful because I remembered how hungry I'd been last time. After this I started to shiver quite badly, so she covered me with a silver blanket and it gradually stopped. I went back into the ward and didn't sleep all night; I was just so excited. I was given my baby to feed first thing the next morning.

I fully intended to breastfeed my baby and had told the midwives. This time, I was so happy to know that I could have my baby so soon. I was in my room in the ward when suddenly the sister from reception appeared in the doorway holding my daughter, as though it was her property. I cannot explain this, but the blood in my veins felt like it froze with my anger. I couldn't believe I could be so unlucky as to have this woman come to teach me about breastfeeding again.

I tried to breastfeed, but had the same problems as last time, sore nipples and worrying about whether the baby was getting enough milk. Sadly, I just couldn't go on and decided to put my daughter on the bottle before I left the hospital.

The sister from reception came and berated me for this, telling me that, "I didn't try very hard," but I kept remembering how unhappy and stressed I was for many weeks last time, and as I now had two children for whom to care, I decided it was best for us all.

(It took me a while, but finally I realised I needed education and help in breast feeding as well, so things eventually changed.)

While I was at the hospital, I went to see a demonstration of a baby being bathed. There were at least 12 other mothers present in the room. The sister from reception was giving the demonstration and came in carrying a sleeping, newborn baby wrapped tightly in a bunny rug. She marched quickly into the room, all authority. On a bed, she had a baby bath ready and all that she would need. Suddenly she took an edge of the rug and flipped the baby out onto the bed. As she pulled on the rug, it unraveled, and the tiny baby rolled out and over. When it landed, its little arms flew up with its fingers stretched out stiff and it screamed loudly and shook in fright.

Every mother in that room gasped in horror and hearing this, the sister from reception looked up at us all and made a joke, "They have to be tough to be born," she said. The baby didn't belong to any mother who was in that room, it was all done for show, but I realised I wasn't the only one intimidated by this midwife, and sadly, not one of us was brave enough to protest at her actions.

When I saw the doctor six weeks later at the follow up visit, he told me he could count on the fingers of one hand the number of women who had done what I had. I really didn't understand, because at that stage, I still didn't know very much. But I couldn't help wondering how many 'natural' births he had ever seen. He told me that hospitals were a monopoly and that he couldn't have made it to the hospital any faster even if he'd flown. I told him I thought the sister from reception was 'rough as bags' and that I had been the only mother in the labour ward the entire time.

But really, I wasn't disappointed about anything anymore. My illusions had fallen away and I knew that he couldn't have cared less about me and that somehow, the entire system was built on deception. The doctors give you the impression that they care about you, but it is the midwives on whom they depend. If the midwives, for whatever reasons, don't care about you, which is often the case, you are just left on your own neglected and negated.

Before he turned up at the birth, I had only seen the doctor once that night, as he appeared in the doorway when I was first admitted into the labour ward, and he hadn't even come into the room. The next time I saw him was some nine hours later when my baby was being born.

I had started to think it was a sort of trick. The doctor depended on the midwives to call him when you are ready to deliver; the waiting is left to the midwives. The system worked for the doctors and midwives, they complemented each other, but often you, the mother, were just left all alone because I found that the midwives didn't care much about you and maybe this was because you were a private patient and they weren't getting the delivery.

In some respects, I thought a mother might be better off in the public system with just the midwives, because at least you knew that there was someone around all the time. You were their responsibility. This is probably why there are fewer Caesareans and fewer complications in the public system, because mothers are less stressed and less left alone, but I don't really know. I felt the midwives were devalued in the private system and became just like a doctor's assistant or handmaiden and maybe they resent this.

I couldn't get over how I'd gained in confidence since my daughter's birth. I felt differently towards my son as well. I had a sense of my own worth as a woman and was beginning to understand that it was my fear and the inability to relax during my first birth that was the trouble. He was stuck in the birth canal, which had become rigid, because of my tension, fear, and the stress that had been inflicted on me by cruel and insensitive hospital practices.

About this time, on television, there would be an occasional program on childbirth. When I watched these, I hated to see women just lying there, their arms lifeless by their sides as they were being 'delivered' as though they had no part in the event. Somehow women have learned that they are helpless when it comes to childbirth and they are not supposed to or allowed to do anything. The doctor or midwife took all the credit, it was as if the mother did nothing.

A doctor once said to me that, "A little knowledge is a dangerous thing." Now I felt that, in my case, "A little knowledge went a long way."

I've also had said to me by a male doctor, "And what medical school did you go to?" as though I, as a mother, who has actually given birth am not supposed to know anything about the process.

However, I was about to understand a lot more when finally, I came across the book "Childbirth Without Fear" written by Dr Grantly Dick-Read.

*Chapter Three*

# A BOOK REVIEW
# "CHILDBIRTH WITHOUT FEAR"

### The Principles and Practice of Natural Childbirth
### by Dr Grantly Dick-Read

**INTRODUCTION**

My first experience of the work of Dr Grantly Dick-Read came inadvertently via a physiotherapist whose classes I attended in 1976 prior to the birth of my second child. Although I had never read Dr Dick-Read's book, through this physiotherapist, I somehow absorbed his teachings. Successfully applying the relaxation and breathing techniques during labour, I gave birth to my daughter as described in the previous chapter.

After her birth, when I was able to get a copy of "Childbirth Without Fear" it was for me a very healing experience to realise that somebody knew what happens in the minds and bodies of women who become very frightened during labour, and that this fear is usually caused by ignorance of the process of birth and loneliness due to lack of support.

Devouring all the scientific knowledge the book contained, I was also impressed by the sympathetic understanding and encouragement Dr Dick-Read gave to women, as I had certainly never experienced anything like this. He had an enormous respect for motherhood and many philosophies about its effect on the world. The book contains numerous scathing criticisms of his fellow medical colleagues and their approach to the women whom they attended. Making too many big waves and enemies within the medical establishment in England, eventually he had to leave and continued practising in South Africa.

It seems to me that the book is largely directed at doctors and midwives, I have never felt it is written solely for mothers, yet mothers embraced it. I feel he is trying to give education on a different way of doing things to promote natural childbirth without injury. In the 1930's and 40's women were mostly giving birth in hospitals with doctors or midwives in attendance, although Britain did have a decreasing culture of home birth for quite some time. Dick-Read wanted women to be educated but it seems to me he only envisaged their giving birth within the hospital setting under the control of doctors and midwives. In his book, he tries to convince medical people to do things differently.

I have several copies of "Childbirth Without Fear". The one I have used the most and is now virtually worn out was published by Har/Row Books, Harper & Row, New York. Copyright 1944, 1953 by Grantly Dick-Read. Copyright 1959 by Jessica Dick-Read. But there are also many other versions.

## DR GRANTLY DICK-READ

Born in Suffolk, England in 1890 he was a Doctor of Medicine, Master of Arts (Natural Science), a Member of the Royal College of Surgeons and a Fellow of the Royal Society of Medicine. He had been writing a book on the facts of childbirth since 1919, and his first book "Natural Childbirth" was published in England in 1932. Ten years later another book entitled "The Revelation of Childbirth" was published. This was again retitled "Childbirth Without Fear" which is the book we know today.

His methods are based on recognising that fear is the enemy of natural childbirth. Fear causes the mother to tense her muscles and in turn this made the pain of childbirth much worse. It also could cause abnormal physical conditions in both the mother and the baby.

Considering that the cervix needs to dilate to 10cms to allow the baby to pass through, he used the words "Tense woman = tense cervix". This meant that if the mother was tense her cervix would also be tense and dilation would be difficult and labour prolonged. If the mother could maintain relaxation with the contractions, her cervix would be able to stretch open more easily and she would experience much less discomfort.

Antenatal classes for expectant mothers were organised by his wife, Jessica, and relaxation and breathing exercises were taught. His patients were encouraged and educated to understand how their uterus worked, its various muscle layers and how they could help themselves during labour. As far as I am aware, no other doctor had ever educated women in this way and as he said, "women now had minds."

Among other aims, he wanted women to know that childbirth could be a joyous and enriching experience. They could destroy fear by education and support, and they could have some control over the course of their labour. He aimed many derogatory comments at his medical colleagues for their inability in realising the magnitude of their responsibility in attending women in childbirth. He wanted women to know the full reward of giving birth and he blamed his colleagues for their medical interferences, which deprived women of these rewards. He said they needed to be interested in both the mental as well as the physical wellbeing of the mother.

At the time he was writing, women were being heavily sedated in labour, they were given drugs and anaesthesia like twilight sleep to counteract the pain of labour. Most mothers were not conscious for the birth of their baby. Dr Dick-Read drew the attention of his colleagues to cerebral palsy, a result of the baby's oxygen starvation at birth. He never withdrew from any controversial issue and seemed to enjoy a good stoush, a result he said from his athletic prowess as a boxer. Dr Dick-Read passed in 1959 aged 69 years.

**Dr Dick-Read and Fear**

As a young doctor in London, he writes how one night he attended a woman in advanced labour. This woman lived in Whitechapel in very poor surroundings. She was accompanied only by a neighbour, but the atmosphere in the room was peaceful and she was quiet and unafraid. As the baby's head was crowning, he wanted to give her chloroform, but she turned her head and refused. He asked her why she wouldn't take it and her reply confounded him when she said it hadn't hurt but also that she didn't think it was meant to.

Sitting with women in labour in hospital, he came to realise that very occasionally there was a calm and peaceful woman who didn't seem to be plagued by the usual agonising pain. This was the catalyst for his starting to investigate the part played by the emotions in labour.

In August 1915 when serving as a doctor at Suvla Bay, Gallipoli during WW1 he gives a moving description of a hideous night attending some 300 injured and dying soldiers on a mud flat. The night was very cold, water was scarce and he administered morphine to those who needed it, there were no boats to take them off the beach.

He describes how, in the stillness, he became aware of utter loneliness. Hearing shots being fired in the distance and the screams of a bayonet charge, he wondered if the enemy had broken through? Would they soon be coming down the hill for him? He was alone and had no companion to ask, he was worn down with apprehension and fear and from this experience he learned how frightening loneliness could be.

Later on, he was at the Somme, at Ypres and many other battles but he says he never suffered as acutely as when he learned the effects of loneliness. He says he would shudder as he went through hospital wards where he knew women were

## Chapter One — Painful Ignorance Sets Off a Learning Curve

labouring behind closed doors without education or support, their minds tortured by fear and their labours prolonged.

It would have caused him great frustration knowing that, within the hospital system, he was powerless to change this. He had developed his own system of treating women through education and support, but he could not intrude or force his views onto others who, it must be surmised, were not as intelligent or forward thinking. He did keep his own statistics for the births he attended and they are still stored in England.

He says he visited his patient when she was first admitted to the labour ward and stayed until he knew she was confident in relaxing with the contractions. He returned for the delivery. There seems to be some misunderstanding that he stayed with women for their entire labour, but I don't think this was the case. Once women understood how to react to the contractions, they were able to continue on their own and his patients mostly never considered or needed any pain relief. He explains that it was always there if required and would never be denied, but that it was hardly ever used.

If a mother was having trouble with her relaxation, he speaks of encouragement and instruction, and where her walls were breaking down, they could be built up again. I wonder if this type of care and understanding is given to women in labour in today's world? During the time Dr Dick Read practised in hospitals, husbands would not have been allowed to be with their wives during labour, nor would any other family members have been admitted. Women would have laboured in isolation. In his own practice, Dr Dick- Read encouraged husbands to be present at the births of their children and to help their wives with back massage.These attitudes to labour, by including the husband, were unheard of at that time.

During WW1 Dr Dick-Read, already suffering from dysentery and fatigue was badly injured when a shell burst almost on top of him. He was left blind in both eyes and could not move his legs, so by hospital ship, he was taken to Malta.

Gradually, as the weeks went by, he started to improve and could see slightly out of one eye. The Blue Sisters ran the hospital and he found great comfort from severe agitation when the Reverend Mother came and sat by him and quietly discussed his progress. Valuing this quiet companionship, which calmed him, he recognised that this was what women needed in labour.

Very ill, he was sent back to London and after recovering he was again returned to France where he sometimes witnessed women giving birth in trenches and by the side of the road. He marvelled at their lack of fear and said often that his own imaginings were much more fearful than anything they were experiencing.

After the war, Dr Dick-Read commenced working with a group of doctors and by 1929 he had a practice in Harley Street, London. He spent hundreds of hours attending women in labour and developing his theories, especially he observed that fear caused the circular muscle fibres of the lower womb to come into action and this constriction caused the pain of childbirth to be greatly worsened. The contractions would still continue with the result that they were trying to pull the cervix open while the fear-induced circular fibres were keeping it tightly closed. Labour would be prolonged.

This is why it is so important for women in labour to know how they can help themselves. Maintaining relaxation with the contractions keeps the cervix in an elastic state making it much easier to stretch open and thereby creating less discomfort.

During the war, when he was suffering acutely from his injuries, an Indian soldier helped Dick-Read by giving instruction in progressive relaxation. This is perhaps where he learned the value of relaxation of the muscles and its practice. It is vitally important during the first stage of labour, because there is no other way to assist the dilation of the cervix except by relaxation. The second stage of labour, when the uterus starts to expel the baby, cannot begin until the cervix has dilated to 10cms. Sometimes, in days past, women were misguidedly told to push from the beginning of labour in the belief that force was the way to get the baby out. This was an exhausting practice for the mother, as pushing against a cervix that is not fully dilated doesn't help at all and will cause bleeding.

**Did His Book Change Anything?**
It certainly made a lot of doctors and obstetricians very angry. As it sold so well in both Britain and the United States there was a lot of jealousy involved and Dick-Read was attacked from many quarters of the medical profession. It seems the women he attended were delighted by his methods and achieved childbirth without fear and pain. They would have helped spread the word, which probably made his jealous colleagues angrier.

In my experience, I have always had pain during childbirth; sometimes so intense it took every ounce of my strength to stay relaxed. As the actual birth became closer, I have entered the amnesic state when the pain is so great and, with relaxation, my body became like a rag doll. Although it looked as though I was asleep, I was consciously aware of everything. Dr Dick-Read explains this phenomenon in his book.

The connection made by Dick-Read about the mother's state of mind, her emotions, and the outcome of her birth had never been addressed before. He was virtually saying to the medical profession that they were causing the problems that women were experiencing because they were too insensitive to realise how the hospital environment, its procedures and systems caused the fear that prevented women from having natural births. It is possible that women who experienced very painful labours and births just accepted that this is how things were and never questioned anything. However, in different circumstances, with different attendants, there may have been a different outcome and no need for their suffering. They probably had no childbirth education and like many women put their trust in doctors and midwives believing they were the experts.

In my own case, had I never become educated after the birth of my first child I am sure I would have been the same, as I accepted everything that was done to me because the explanations sounded feasible, but upon further learning and experience I realised the mistakes due to lack of care of the mother's emotions during labour. When giving birth in hospitals, women are isolated from each other; we have no way of knowing what has happened to another woman unless she shares her experiences.

Dr Dick-Read abhorred episiotomy, a deliberate cut made with scissors in the mother's perineum, the area between the vagina and the anus, to make the vaginal opening larger. Some doctors think it is better not to allow the perineum to tear, as a cut is easier to stitch and heals better than a tear. In natural childbirth, if a woman is encouraged and knows to relax her pelvic floor, if she is getting plenty of oxygen through her breathing and is not forced to violently push, the tissues can expand and there is no need for tears or episiotomy. The baby is born by uterine force alone and, in my experience, the perineum is not even involved. Whereas, violently pushing down into the rectum actually hardens the perineum. One midwife even said to me it would be better if mothers were told to push up, not down.

Some hospital attendants would never have any experience of these methods and many doctors and midwives wouldn't think twice about cutting an episiotomy. Bilateral episiotomies are even cut in some instances and women often report that episiotomies can be very painful and sometimes take a long time to heal and some never do.

A doctor told me in the 1980's, when I mentioned rooming in, that I had no right to complain about anything in the hospital, I was alive and I had a live baby, what more did I want? This was his criterion, which told me he wasn't interested in the experience of the mother and anything done by medical attendants was acceptable. It is very probable that this type of attitude existed in Dick-Read's time. Their profession was one of prestige and power and they didn't like being challenged.

By criticising his medical colleagues in his book, it was almost as though Dr Dick-Read was sending a veiled warning message to women that things might not be as we think. He was introducing new thoughts and encouraging women through education that they had some control over their labours. This was in an era when women had little influence or power worldwide.

His book certainly drew attention to himself and his beliefs and would have attracted a lot of clients to his practice. Proud of their medical training, I don't think obstetricians and doctors would have wanted to change their practices. If they read his book, they were probably antagonistic towards him for treading on their territory and authority.

With the doctor's presence, midwifery has been eroded and many midwives would now only be able to practice in the hospital environment. This is probably very frustrating for them as a profession, but it is something they have learned to accept. The only time I ever had a midwife stay with me was at my home birth.

**Specific Chapters**
Some chapters from the book are: The Pain of Labour; Anatomy & Physiology; Low Threshold of Pain Interpretation; Fear; Diet; Labour; Hypnosis; The Conduct of Labour; Emergency Childbirth; Breast Feeding and Rooming In; The Husband and Childbirth; and Antenatal Education just to name a few.

Despite the year in which it was first published, there is a lot of information that is still relevant. Some of his writing might seem dated to our ears as words change and people have different forms of expression. There is also certain romanticism and warmth that I think some women will appreciate. Interestingly, I have never met anyone, whether doctor, midwife or mother who has read it.

On one occasion when I spoke about it with a group of student-midwives they accused me of being idealistic. It is not difficult to understand their attitude, they are what they are taught and they see the results. Alternatively, if they were taught differently and adopted different attitudes, they would see very different results.

**A Word About Pain**
Having only experienced natural childbirth through being educated, I have a learned response to the pain of contractions. They don't frighten me; they are something to be dealt with because I understand that they are trying to pull open the cervix, to pull it up over the baby's head. If our cervix was already open, as the baby grew bigger in the womb, it would just fall out. So, our cervix needs to stretch out from being closed to 10cms to allow the baby to come down into the birth canal and be born into the outside world.

If you have read my story in Chapter One of the birth of my first child, I can distinctly remember that I was at home for several hours before my husband and I went to the hospital. During that time, I was very aware of the uterus contracting, and as a first-time mother, I had no fear or apprehension of what was ahead. The only vague instruction I received was from a small book that said, "You must relax, " and that was all. Not much to go on, but relax is what I did.

My uterus was doing all the right things, and following the instruction to relax, in my innocence, I was simply allowing everything to happen unhindered. When my mother-in- law came to sit with me, I think she was amazed at my composure and she really thought I wasn't doing anything. Yet I was feeling all the sensations of labour, without fear, and I was dilating beautifully.

Some hours later, upon arrival at the hospital, my husband and I waited for an hour in the waiting room while the staff was at dinner. This was in 1975. Nobody welcomed us, the midwife in the reception area just told us to sit and wait and she disappeared. The whole area was unattended. We were there alone and it was at this time that I started to feel the contractions as painful. Not long afterwards upon finally being examined internally, they were shocked to find I was 8cms dilated. However, not receiving any support and being ignorant of how to help myself, I succumbed to fear and terror from this good beginning.

**About Ballerinas**
Perhaps it is pertinent to mention here that Dr Dick-Read said he often wished that ballerinas and Centre Court Wimbledon "types" would cease to come to him because they so often had a lot of trouble. He said they had magnificent physiques but were often nervous and highly strung like a lot of athletes. They relied on themselves for success. When he realised how sensitive they were, he used a more understanding approach, and, once educated, these women became excellent subjects for natural childbirth and were a pleasure for him to attend.

Having learned classical ballet from the age of eight years, I guess I might fall into this category. Both in England and Australia, I had a professional career in dancing. Those who have been trained in classical ballet will know that from an early age we need to remember many steps. You cannot dance with a piece of paper in your hands, everything needs to be committed to memory. Probably like many trained dancers, I can actually remember dances I learned when I was eight years old. My secretarial skills also helped me to record my experiences.

Sensitivity is not necessarily a weakness. It can help us to have insight into other people's experiences, and understanding others can be a great strength, especially in childbirth. And here also, I would like to address what the midwife told me during labour with my first baby, namely that because I was fit, and had been a dancer, I would have 'nice, tight muscles'. I don't believe that this is the case. A toned muscle is not necessarily a tight muscle, it has the ability to relax when the mind tells it to. So just because you are a fit person doesn't mean you are 'tight' or more likely to have problems. If a mother has 'tight' muscles in labour, it is probably because she has become very frightened and this is usually due to lack of education and lack of support.

I was still very fit in my four, subsequent births, but by then I knew how to keep relaxed with the contractions even though I rarely received any encouragement or instruction from midwives or doctors. To my mind, whether fit or unfit, giving birth naturally depends more on the mother's ability to keep calm and relaxed. While fitness is desirable, I feel it has little to do with the outcome of labour.

During labour, if Dr Dick-Read gave instruction and support to the women he attended, and they were educated in classes run by his wife, their minds were probably free from fear and greatly at ease. They had been given both the education and support needed to have their babies naturally.

## Natural Childbirth and Hypnosis

It was suggested to Dr Dick-Read that by reading his book, women in America and Germany were being hypnotised by him in 12 different languages all over the world. It was a preposterous suggestion and greatly amused him. He explains that it was the natural childbirth teaching that was helping women, replacing their ignorance with understanding and simple techniques to help themselves. He wanted the principles and procedures of natural childbirth to be "entirely alienated from the conscious employment of hypnotism."

## In Conclusion

Dr Dick-Read believed that many of the unforeseen complications of labour, such as interference, haemorrhage, tissue injury and psychopathy in the mother, and anoxia, respiratory failure and exhaustion in the infant, were caused by lack of education, lack of support or medical mismanagement during labour, which all contributed to fear in the mother.

If women want to experience natural childbirth, they will need to be educated in how to help themselves knowing that relaxation combined with effective breathing and perseverance are their strength. If they can find attendants who are sympathetic and helpful, they will be very fortunate.

Good quality antenatal care was imperative for women and this included care of both the mind and the body. Good midwifery was essential to protect the woman in labour from fear-producing words and actions.

The status of women at the time his book was written was not very high, but he knew this and he also knew that, in the future, this would change. There are probably many issues that could be debated, but as a man of his time, I feel he did everything he could to bring about better outcomes for mothers and their babies.

*Chapter Four*

# A BOOK REVIEW
# "NO TIME FOR FEAR"

### by Dr Grantly Dick-Read

First published in 1955 this book describes the journey taken by Dr Dick-Read around South Africa to document the births of primitive women. For years he had taught his method of natural childbirth to "unnatural" women and now he wanted to compare these methods with the birth customs of those women who lived nearest to nature.

Accompanied by his wife Jessica, his secretary and a young native boy they set out in a specially built caravan on August 18th 1953 on a journey of some 6,000 miles through Africa from Johannesburg to Mombasa.

It was a challenge for him to prove his beliefs that his medical colleagues were misinterpreting the laws of nature and implementing modern scientific methods to hide not only the pain of childbirth, but also their failure to understand its cause.

There were many difficulties to overcome throughout the journey. The roads were hazardous, especially in the mountains. There were elephants, lions and giant ants to be guarded against as well as the ever-present threat of mechanical breakdowns.

The information he gathered and his observations of the

childbirth customs at that time were as follows:

The African woman, when attended in her village, was never left alone. She was well instructed in the course of labour by old women in whom she had complete confidence.

Between 94% and 98% in different tribes had normal, natural births. Their mistakes were tragedies for they did not have the ability to understand irregularities. But their customs did not allow the acts and interferences, which account for over 60% of maternal morbidity in the white man's countries.

Every tribe and village had a profound respect for the afterbirth.

No child was separated from its mother until the afterbirth was born.

The babies were fed at the breast. The natives believed the mother's spirit flowed through her milk to nourish the child with the love that made strong men and fertile women.

The children were carried securely in wraps and knew no loneliness or absence of a mother's care. Grandmothers were also able to breast-feed the children.

Dr Dick-Read believed in 1953 that within 20 years of his journey these customs would have disappeared. He says, "There is so much wisdom, yet so much ignorance of the reasons why they are so wise." The Africans had learned quickly from the white man, but did the white man learn in his turn? He believed that if the wisdom of the primitive African woman was combined with the understanding of the white people, the trials and tribulations of childbirth would be reduced to a negligible figure.

He says, "There will always be abnormalities in all forms of reproduction throughout the realms of nature, but the complications of pathological childbirth are few compared with the man-made troubles that emerge through his failure to understand the simple physiological mechanism and its demands."

In his ability to understand people Dr Dick-Read possessed a unique quality and whether he is writing of a Leper colony or of the pride of old women who have borne 15 children, he conveys great warmth and simplicity and writes of his feelings from the heart.

He was 63 years of age when he undertook this journey through Africa and one cannot help but admire his great courage and determination in his efforts to make the experience of childbirth one of monumental joy and achievement for women everywhere.

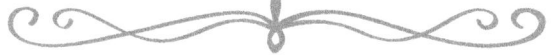

*Chapter Five*

# DIFFERENT HOSPITAL – SIMILAR STRESSES

In July 1977, at 30 years of age, I gave birth to our third child. We both thought this baby would complete our family.

Earlier that year, we had watched a television program based on the work of Dr Frederick Leboyer, who was a French doctor specialising in gynaecology and obstetrics. He advocated a peaceful environment for the birth of a baby, devoid of bright lights and loud noises, to prevent emotional and physical distress. Leboyer's book first published in Paris in 1974 was entitled "Birth Without Violence".

The baby was placed on the mother's stomach and the umbilical cord was not cut immediately as it was still a source of oxygen. After it had drained of blood, it was cut. The baby was able to make its first movements supported in a bath that allowed it to stretch its limbs for the first time, weightless, without any stress.

Watching the TV program, I understood that this type of sensitivity towards a newborn baby would also be of benefit to its mother. There was a Childbirth Education Association near my suburb and I had become a member. They advertised a meeting with a panel of doctors and midwives to discuss this book and film, and so my husband and I attended.

From the discussions, I learned of a private hospital not too far away from where we lived offering this type of birth. Upon making enquiries, I was given the names of doctors who attended births at this hospital and we made an appointment to see one.

He was enthusiastic about this way of welcoming the baby. At our first interview I was able to tell him what had happened to me previously and how I practiced natural childbirth using the methods of Dr Grantly Dick-Read. I actually had Dick-Read's book with me and I said to the doctor that I couldn't understand why others hadn't adopted his methods.

This doctor examined my pregnant tummy and all was well, that was it, there was no need to remove my clothes or conduct an internal examination, for which I was very relieved. Over the coming months, I went for my antenatal visits until the birth was imminent.

My baby seemed again to be quite big and at an antenatal visit the day prior to the birth, the doctor said my cervix was wide open and three fingers dilated (around 3cms), although I wasn't yet in labour. This was the first internal examination I'd had with this doctor. I asked him about shaving off my pubic hair and he said there was no need.

The following morning, I discovered a show of brown mucous and rang the doctor. Upon arriving at the surgery, he again examined me and I had now dilated to 4 fingers (around 4cms). After this examination, once I started to walk, I felt contractions begin, so prepared for the trip to the hospital.

As I believed this would be my last experience in childbirth, and the hospital had rooming-in, we booked a private room so I would be able to have my baby with me all the time. The Nursing Mothers' Association, which I had discovered was in our area, had meetings and as I really wanted to breast feed I'd joined. I found their books and meetings very helpful although, compared to some of these women, I was lacking in confidence and feeling a bit of a failure. Nipple preparation by massaging, rolling and gently pulling

## Chapter Five — Different Hospital —Similar Stresses

out my nipples was something I had been doing for many weeks as I was hoping to avoid previous problems.

My husband needed a haircut and so we called in at a shopping centre on the way to hospital. As I was heavily pregnant, I received a few strange looks. We found a hairdresser and I sat in the waiting area reading a magazine. I mentioned to the female hairdresser that I was in early labour, but it was early stages. She just smiled and understood. The poor male hairdresser, who was cutting my husband's hair was beside himself. He constantly looked over at me and his eyes were popping out of their sockets. He seemed relieved when we were leaving.

It was about 1:00pm when we arrived at the hospital. No pubic shaves or enemas were required and I was able to wear my own nightie. In my two previous labours, once contractions were regular, my bowels had moved of their own accord and this time, that's what happened again.

Some time ago, a midwife explained to me that it is good to have an empty bowel as it means more room for the baby and with the expulsive action of the uterus in second stage, you avoid having a bowel motion at the same time as the baby is being born.

Over the next few hours, my husband and I sat in the beautiful grounds of this hospital and, as it was wintertime, it was pleasant being in the warm sunshine. Later in the afternoon we came into the labour room, a midwife gave me an internal examination and I was 7cm dilated. Breathing and relaxing with each one, it was hard work for me; the contractions were very strong but not yet close enough together.

At 8 pm I was 9cm dilated. The midwife suggested she would pop the membranes if I wished her to, but it was to be my choice. We decided to wait an hour, as my membranes had never ruptured on their own in both previous births, they'd always been broken and we were hoping things would be different this time.

At one stage, a midwife told us the baby was transverse; this was news to me, as the doctor had never mentioned it. If I'd been a first-time mother, I can imagine the midwife saying this might have frightened me; I just said to myself, 'as long as I keep relaxed, everything will be alright.' But I thought to myself, it was very insensitive.

Although I was in a private hospital, I found very little warmth or attention from the midwives. They didn't appear to be rushed off their feet. Perhaps it's because they are all trained the same way, and perhaps I had been expecting something different. There was nothing special about the room, and I wish I hadn't gone onto the bed so early. Sitting up straight, supported by pillows, I was getting a numb derriere.

At 9:15pm I could not make a decision about my membranes. How I wished the doctor was there. Once again, I was caught up in this tense situation of waiting for the doctor. Did he know what was happening? My husband, venting his frustration, said to the midwife at one stage, "Does he even know we're here?" The midwife informed us that she had rung the doctor and he was on his way, but it was up to us to choose whether or not to rupture the membranes.

Deciding I couldn't wait any longer, the midwives broke the membranes, and one of them said they were like canvas. As the warm water flowed out of me, a flood of tears also came and I think I shed a lot of tension. How I hated this interaction with the midwives and the to-ing and fro-ing between them and the doctor. My antenatal care had been with the doctor and once again, there was this impersonal communication with people I had never met before. The midwives had a certain power and the doctor needed them to be there, but I hated being in the middle of it.

The contractions were now very intense. When they ruptured the membranes, I'd had to slide down flat on the bed with my legs apart and once the water had gone, I felt the baby slide further down into the birth canal. I can only think that by sitting up so straight in the bed, I might have actually prolonged things.

Finally, the doctor arrived and as he came into the room,

he immediately asked the midwife to turn down the lights. How I wish we'd had the courage to ask earlier, as the dim light was a tremendous relief and assisted me to keep on with my inner relaxation. He told me to lie back against the pillows and close my eyes. After an internal examination, he said there was no cervix left. The contractions were fierce and before long I started to feel the pressure from my uterus as it began pressing out the baby.

Neither forcing nor hindering whatever the uterus was doing, I just remained passive, waiting. With each contraction I could feel my abdominal muscles coming into action. Being very sleepy I was aware that the doctor lifted my arm up and let it drop onto the bed. Each time it fell as though it was lifeless. He was demonstrating my state of relaxation to the two midwives who were present, but somehow, I don't think they appreciated it. My husband was very encouraging, telling me I was going great.

At least I was on the same page as the doctor. One of the midwives said to him that I needed to start bearing down with the contractions. Even in my amnesic state, I said, "No". This was because my uterus was already doing that, but I'm sure these women were only used to taking over and seeing mothers with their legs up, holding their breath and being told to forcefully push down to get their baby out.

They simply don't realise that relaxation, even in second stage labour, assists the uterus to function and extra force is unnecessary as it makes the mother tense. If she has to hold her breath and bear down, she cuts off her oxygen. Having to hold up her legs at the same time is a ridiculous position for a birthing woman, sometimes referred to as "the stranded beetle" position.

After my saying 'no', the doctor said to the midwives, "This woman has a very strong character and we must respect that." Feeling very uncomfortable about this situation I just kept on with the relaxation and with each expulsive contraction, I felt the gradual expansion of the vagina. My husband and two midwives were still in the room and at one stage the doctor went out the door for a short period of time.

The birth was imminent, but as I am so quiet during labour, I think that only I knew it. As the doctor came back into the room, I saw the surprised look on his face, as the baby's head had crowned. Quickly, a large mirror was placed at the end of the bed so I could watch the birth. How marvellous this was, as I had never had it before. It completely took me out of myself and I watched in awe as the baby's head passed through my vagina.

With the next contraction, the baby was born and I had the most overwhelming sense of relief. I heard my husband say, "Darling, it's a boy." It was 10:42 pm.

In just a short while, in the dim light, my baby was placed onto my stomach. He had given a soft cry as he was born. Looking in the mirror, I could see the cord coming out of me; we were still attached to each other. Feelings of joy, relief and peace came over me. When the cord had finished pulsating, my husband cut it with the assistance of the doctor. The afterbirth must have been delivered, but I don't recall even seeing it. I marvelled at this new, little one, so different from the others.

Our baby was then placed in his first bath, where my husband held him and allowed him to move freely suspended in the warm water for some 10 minutes. It was then time for me to put the baby to the breast, which he took without any problem. When they weighed him, he was 9lbs 6 ozs (4.25kg). Slipping through as he did, I didn't need any stitches.

It had seemed like a long labour and I stayed at the hospital for about four days. Breast-feeding wasn't a problem and I enjoyed being with this new little boy very much. Everything had gone well and I was grateful to this doctor for believing in me.

My physiotherapist told me a story about certain maternity hospitals in the 1940's. Being the mother of six children, she said at that time children were not allowed even to visit their mother in the hospital. Mothers had to stay in hospital for two weeks and were often not even allowed out of bed for some days.

## Chapter Five — Different Hospital –Similar Stresses

It was the same for her, as all her children had been born in hospital. Her husband would bring the older children to see their mother, but they could only stand outside on the footpath. She said it was so distressing for her seeing her older children all lined up crying their eyes out as they waved to her. In turn, crying her eyes out, she waved back to them from an upstairs window. At least some progress has been made since those days. But you can't help wondering what type of people, even in those times, would make up rules like this.

Breast-feeding still caused me some problems, with cracked nipples and a breast infection. This baby sucked very strongly; but I managed to breastfed him for six months. To overcome the breast infection, whenever I could, I would get in the shower after a feed and manually express whatever milk was left in my breast. In a short while, everything settled down, I didn't want to give up this time.

For the next eight years, we brought up our children and I thought that our family was now complete. Sometimes I thought it would be wonderful for our children to have the joy of a younger brother or sister in their lives, to help care for it and watch it grow. I wondered if we had finished our family after all.

These thoughts did become reality, and so after eight years, I was happy to be expecting another baby. I was 37 years of age, still fit and healthy.

*Chapter Six*

# A VERY DIFFICULT LESSON

Eight years after the birth of our third child, my husband and I decided it would be lovely to have a child to share with our three children, who were now about 10, 9 and 8 years of age. They would have a younger brother or sister who they could grow to love. Being 37 years of age, I was lucky to be in good health and so in due course I became pregnant. We decided to go to the doctor we had seen previously and the same private hospital. This doctor was still offering the Leboyer method of welcoming the baby and this had been a very happy experience for us.

There were a lot of new books about childbirth and one of them encouraged mothers to give birth actively by standing up, kneeling, squatting or on all fours. It seemed that any position was preferable to a mother being on her back. Moving around during labour gave her freedom to follow her natural instincts. Having purchased a copy of this book I simply couldn't apply any of it to myself. But I thought that, if adopting any of these positions helped a woman in labour to relax and helped her to cope with the contractions, then I could see the benefits.

As I had walked for some time during my last two labours, I already knew the value of keeping upright and not getting on a bed too early. But when I looked at the pictures in this book, the women on all fours were being delivered from behind; I didn't think this was very "active." Although I was still very fit, I knew that during the amnesic stage of labour, when you are relaxing with the enormous contractions; the endorphins and the intense pain make you very limp and sleepy, and all I would be able to do was be supported on a bed. This book went into my bookcase and I never gave it any further thought.

## An Introduction to Homebirth

In my area, there were several women having homebirths. They started a group, which was advertised in the local paper, and as I was pregnant, I went along to their meetings. Their efforts to give birth in their own home impressed me. Homebirth midwives also came to the meetings and I enjoyed speaking with them. Sometimes I spoke about natural childbirth, Dr Dick-Read, and the need to be educated in breathing and relaxation to avoid fear in labour.

The group listened to me and empathised over my hospital births, but I don't think they were impressed by my knowledge. There was a "hippie" element to homebirth and this never worried me, but I did think that many of the women placed too much responsibility on the midwife without educating themselves. The women I met were well read, politically astute and extremely keen on good nutrition; I learned a lot from them. Some smoked, which concerned me, but on the other hand, without exception, all breast fed their babies. Sometimes I went far afield to attend different meetings, but somehow, I still couldn't see myself having a homebirth.

## First Time Mothers

Sometimes, people will say that labour with a first baby is slower, or is the cause of more complications. Yet I met two women who were planning homebirths and whose first babies were born in the car on the way to hospital. I can only think that their labouring in the home environment was free of stress and so they, unknowingly, dilated very quickly.

## Chapter Six — A Very Difficult Lesson

There is really no reason for a first-time mother to be afraid that her labour will be slower or more painful. Once again, I feel that if she is practising relaxation and breathing with the contractions, she will dilate effectively. But hearing other people's negative opinions about first time mothers could cause a woman to become fearful, and this is the problem, which can be overcome by education and support.

Everything was ready for this birth. My three children were old enough to be included and present, if they wished, when the baby was being born; a regular occurrence at the hospital. There was a separate playroom and television for the children too. When I went into labour, we thought it would be good not to go to the hospital too early.

The previous day I had an antenatal visit with the doctor and he gave me an internal examination and said the birth would be happening very soon and the baby's head was right down in the pelvis. During this visit, I thought it strange that he showed me a lot of photographs of women in labour. They were leaning over beanbags on the floor, and in various positions such as kneeling, squatting and on all fours. Most were being delivered from behind.

It slowly dawned on me that he wanted me to adopt these positions for my birth. Recognising this concept from the book I had read, I said to him, very clearly, that I didn't want to do any of this. My main objective was to stay relaxed and I just wanted to recline on the bed supported by pillows. He looked at me intently and unfortunately, I didn't realise how committed he was to this type of active birth.

As I was at my due date, I went into labour the following day. The children and everything needed to be organised and so I was upright and mobile nearly all day. Having a shower before we left for the hospital, I was worried I'd left it too late, as the contractions were very strong. In the car, I was hanging on for dear life; I'd forgotten how strong the contractions could be.

We arrived at the hospital at 4:30pm and found out I was six centimetres dilated. There was a soft, comfortable chair in the room so I just sat in this, making it very easy for me to stay relaxed. At 6:00pm, I was fully dilated. After the midwife examined me, I stayed on the bed and rested against the pillows.

My husband and two of my children were in the room, while the youngest stayed in the TV room. The doctor came very quickly and I was grateful that everything was turning out so well. My second stage contractions had been going on since the last examination by the midwife, although once again, as I am so quiet and practising relaxation, it is difficult for others to tell. But I knew the baby was almost ready to be born and I was very happy and relieved that the doctor was there.

When he came into the room, he said how marvellous this all was. He crossed the floor to the far corner of the room and one of the midwives helped him into a green gown and gloves. He hadn't examined me; I suppose maybe not wanting to do this in front of my children. Being now very amnesic and reclining against supporting pillows, I must have looked as though I was asleep.

It is difficult for me to explain what happened next, but suddenly I heard him shout from the corner, "You're in the worst, possible position you can be in, get on your side."

Trying to rouse myself, I didn't really comprehend what he was saying, so I never moved. Yet again, he shouted from the corner, "Get on your side." There was now a midwife standing either side of me, both had their arms folded. Neither made a move and I didn't want to move, so I didn't.

What was happening? Maybe the doctor thought I wasn't coping and the pain was too great for me. I was in second stage labour, but there wasn't any need for me to change position.

Again, from the corner of the room, he shouted emphatically, "Get on your side."

## Chapter Six — A Very Difficult Lesson

The room was filled with tension and anxiously my husband said, "Try it, darling, try it."

I was in utter confusion. There was no need for me to move, I wasn't in any distress, I was happy as I was and I knew my baby was about to be born.

Seeing the faces of my two children, and sensing the tension in the room, I realised I had to do something. Somehow, I managed to lever myself up, pressing down on my hands and while in mid-air I quickly turned over to my left landing with a thud on my left side onto the bed. It was the worst possible thing I could have done. My uterus went crazy as my big tummy hit the bed. I guess I was trying to keep the peace for everybody's sake.

Once on my side, I couldn't see anyone in the room. All I could see was the lower part of the midwife on my left, and how her arms were both folded across her stomach. Now my uterus violently contracted and it drove hard, expelling the baby. I think the membranes ruptured as they were still intact. I'd never experienced such pain, so it was an enormous effort for me to stay relaxed and in control.

Quickly came another contraction with the same violence and no break in between, this one pushed out the baby's head. The midwife said to me, "Put your hand down and touch your baby's head."

Where was it? I was disorientated, not knowing where the head was located. Finally, I found my right buttock and let my hand go down, gently exploring where I thought the baby's head would be. The pain was the worst I had ever felt in my life but knowing my children were in the room, I stayed in control. Again, my uterus gave a huge contraction and the baby was born. Divorced from the entire room, I hardly knew what was happening. From behind me, my husband said, "Darling, it's a little boy."

The doctor was also behind me on my right and trying to put the baby on my tummy. But I was still on my left side and had on my nightie. Somehow, I moved onto my back to receive this little baby and my husband helped me take off my nightie to allow the baby to have contact with my skin. It was all very awkward. At that point, my third child ran into the room and I said to him that he had a little brother. This somehow brought me back to earth. My husband cut the cord and we went through the bathing and took photos with the children.

Breast-feeding was no problem afterward, as the baby was with me. The doctor visited me every day for the four days I stayed in the hospital. When I returned home, I knew there was something wrong with me, but I didn't know what it was. The baby was thriving, but my mind felt as though it was in pieces. Still needing to run the house, get meals and take children to and from school and sporting events, I didn't have much time to think about how I felt.

The homebirth women were very supportive, visited and brought me cards, as did the women from the Childbirth Education Association, although I think some of them sensed I was withdrawn and quiet. It is hard to know how to describe this feeling, but I think I felt agitated and found it difficult to relax.

**A New Understanding**
After speaking about this birth to various people, the homebirth group asked me to travel to a meeting and speak about my latest birth experience. This was probably about six months later. It was while I was telling my story that I said, "Of course, I didn't see anything as I was on my side." Like a clap of thunder, I realised my trouble.

My expectation had been that I would again see the birth in a mirror, but I had neglected to specify this to the doctor. I simply didn't realise that his methods had changed and he was now so taken up with active birth. Clearly, I had told him of my wishes to be reclining on pillows on the bed, but this is anathema to passionate proponents of active birth who want to see mothers in any position other than on their back.

Becoming closer to the women in the homebirth group as they were so supportive, I was speaking with one woman and I

## Chapter Six — A Very Difficult Lesson

mentioned to her how the doctor had virtually yelled at me, several times, from the corner of the room to get on my side. There was really no need, as I was calm and quiet and happy as I was. Also, the midwives never moved or offered any support at all while physically, I had to find a way to turn on my side. And, even if they had disagreed with the doctor's actions, they probably wouldn't be able to say anything anyway.

As a homebirth mother, this woman looked at me and incredulously she said, "But why didn't you just tell him to piss off?"

Stunned, I couldn't stop thinking about this.

She added, "In those minutes when he was yelling at you, you would have had to work through all your conditioning to make a decision. This was enormously stressful when you were just about to give birth."

It was so true; and now I was questioning all that, and what a shattered mess I was. To sort myself out, I started nine months of therapy, without drugs. Going once a week, the therapist made me think for myself. Her mantra seemed to be, "And what do you think you can do about that?"

There were also some other issues in my life that I needed to sort out.

My husband saw my pain and tried to understand, and gradually, life settled down. Our little boy was growing fast, and I breastfed him for 17 months and I really enjoyed it too. But we hadn't realised how alone he would be going through childhood on his own. We decided to have another child, but this time the birth would be at home.

*Chapter Seven*

# HOMEBIRTH

Experiences in childbirth always greatly impacted my life. The fact that women were suffering unnecessarily aroused in me a strong sense of injustice. Many didn't know the value of childbirth education or how to help themselves during labour. Although they might get some education through the hospital antenatal classes, it was geared to making them dependent on doctors and midwives. It certainly wasn't the same as education in natural childbirth, which helped a woman to understand the birth process and have more control during labour.

Meeting with homebirth mothers and midwives was a wonderful outlet for me, simply because everyone was interested in childbirth and babies, but not necessarily natural childbirth. Some homebirth women I met were quite averse to hearing my views on childbirth education, especially if I mentioned Dr Grantly Dick-Read, as he was a doctor and a male. I tried to say, 'but you wouldn't want to throw the baby out with the bath water just because he was a man?' What I meant was that it would be a shame to ignore everything that he had learned and written from attending women during labour. Also, he was super sensitive to women's feelings and needs.

At 39 years of age, I was in good health, so we planned a homebirth for our fifth and last child. Finding a homebirth midwife was important, somebody with whom we both felt comfortable. Thankfully there were several women in our area having homebirths and I met one of the midwives who was attending them. We had a meeting in our home and she asked me to write down what I expected of her. This is what I wrote:

"I just want to let my baby come out into my hands or onto the bed and I want to pick it up myself and put it on my tummy. I will be semi-reclining and watching the birth in a mirror."

I remember she said to us, words to the effect that she would just take a back seat.

Homebirth didn't frighten me. I knew from previous births I was able to keep calm and relax and breathe with the contractions of labour and this was how to avoid complications. Two of my friends, both mothers, were eager to help at the birth, and it would be a very family-orientated experience for everyone. My midwife visited me regularly throughout the pregnancy. These visits were very relaxed and not at all rushed and she provided us with a list of the requirements we would need, which posed no problem as we just about had everything anyway. My GP also gave me antenatal care and wasn't worried that I was having a homebirth.

## The Day of our Homebirth

It had been a hot, January day; labour probably started around 5:00 pm and was firmly establishing itself by 8:00 pm. The contractions were strong and regular and I had telephoned everybody involved. Staying upright, I completed some household chores and had a shower. My children were excited and my helpers had arrived.

I found leaning forward over the kitchen bench was a good place to relax until the contractions passed.

Around 10:30pm, contractions were five minutes apart and about midnight, my midwife arrived and examined me. My cervix was 6cms dilated with intact membranes. There was no pain during this examination and as I was relaxing all my muscles, she said my cervix was soft and stretchy, but very sutured.

No longer feeling that I wanted to walk around, I moved to the bedroom and onto a reclining chair that we had borrowed. It was very supportive and the ideal position for me. My fifth child seemed to be a big baby, and I was conscious that my abdomen was a bit pendulous. My midwife and I felt that this was the best supportive position. The baby's position was noted as Right Occipito Posterior. I knew if I maintained my relaxation, this position posed no problem.

I had spoken with her about my previous birth and the active birth concept. I said I couldn't understand it because women on all fours didn't seem to be actively involved in the actual birth, they were delivered from behind. I also said I didn't think it would be any good for me because if I was on all fours, the weight of the baby in my abdomen would be hanging, dragging me down. She agreed with me and said she thought it was better to keep the baby's head on the cervix.

Things hotted up pretty fast, and by 1:20am my uterus started to press the baby out. My midwife had told me this pressure from the uterus starts when the baby's head is low down and onto the pelvic floor. However, I never used any extra force or effort, only as much pressure as my uterus told me and when it told me. The membranes ruptured by themselves and the amniotic fluid was nice and clear. The contractions that I was now experiencing were huge, and instinctively I put my hands under my tummy for support.

I would breathe calmly at the start of a contraction, but as it reached its peak, I would pant more quickly in and out through my mouth to get extra oxygen. As it subsided, it was just normal, calm breathing and I always felt more relaxation as I exhaled through my mouth. This is the way I breathed throughout labour. During a contraction, my tummy would rise up and be rock hard, I knew this was pulling open my cervix.

It is difficult to speak of the pain of a contraction. At this stage, I was consumed by it, but it comes, reaches a huge peak and then subsides. At least for me. Sometimes I would think,

'How could I ever explain this to others?' because it is so intense.

As the uterus pressed out, around 1:50am I felt the gradual expansion of the birth canal as the baby's head came on view and crowned. This meant the very top of its head was at the entrance to the birth canal. With the next contraction, the baby's head passed through with pressure from the uterus, and it had lots of black hair.

There was a sensation of stinging as all the tissues around the vagina expand, but I never felt it was extreme, just like if you open your mouth really wide. Once the baby's head passes through, the sensation quickly disappears. I put my hands down to touch its head and it slightly swivelled itself around, still inside me. Everyone was so supportive. My hips were aching like mad, but I couldn't change position and I just put up with it.

Finally, at 1:55am, the baby slid out and I scooped it up. I was pretty overcome with emotion, as when the baby is finally born, the relief is so great and the pain is gone. You just can't believe you've done it. I didn't need any stitches. I could have expelled the placenta sooner, but we were all taken up with the excitement. Finally, at 3:15 am, we put some traction on the cord and the placenta came out, "Complete and large". It had obviously just been sitting in the birth canal.

The baby was a little girl (we'd had no prior knowledge), something we had hoped for, and she weighed 9lbs 4ozs. (4.196 kg). Our midwife stayed overnight and visited regularly over the next two weeks.

Although, for months, I'd prepared my nipples by massaging them and pulling them out, I still had the usual cracked nipples, but I had plenty of milk. Eventually, my midwife advised me to take off my nursing bra altogether.

It was a hot summer and too hot and humid in my nursing bra, what with nursing pads and moisture, the air needed to circulate around my breasts to heal the cracks. So, I walked around braless in t-shirts and singlets, and changed when they became too damp. But it worked and the cracks healed. I also had warm showers after feeding and expressed the excess milk.

As this was my last child, I fed her for 2 years and 10 months. It was no trouble. For probably the final year, it was just for comfort, morning and night.

A man of his time, I don't think Dr Grantly Dick-Read ever thought of women taking the responsibility of childbirth on themselves. He wrote largely to bring awareness to doctors and midwives about the necessity of educating mothers and providing emotional support in order to prevent fear from invading the mother's mind during labour. He tried to educate them on how fear affected women in childbirth. He tried to make them aware of the causes of this fear.

I remember reading Dr Dick Read's description of the separation of the afterbirth. He said the mother's physical reaction, upon hearing her baby, was a natural stimulus that closed off the blood supply to the placenta and caused it to separate. You have to wonder if today, there is any medical person who would believe this.

Having missed out on seeing the birth of my fourth child, I was overcome as I watched this birth in a mirror that we set up. If she wishes it, there really is no other way for a mother to see the birth. Dr Dick-Read advocated having a mirror for the mother and I found it helped me and was a distraction from the pain.

During the birth, my midwife steeped towelling nappies in hot water, wrung them out, tested them on her cheek and placed these hot towels right across my genital area. They felt amazing and greatly assisted my ability to relax. My helpers had everything washed and hanging on the clothesline before they left. At this point my husband and I held our new baby in her first bath and soon, everyone was asleep except me. I was so excited that everything had gone well.

Around 6:00am, just after sunrise, I was feeding the baby and when she'd finished, I walked outside in the fresh air and saw the elderly man next door in his garden. Our new daughter was wrapped in a lightweight bunny rug and I said to him that I'd had her last night. He happily congratulated me and my little bundle.

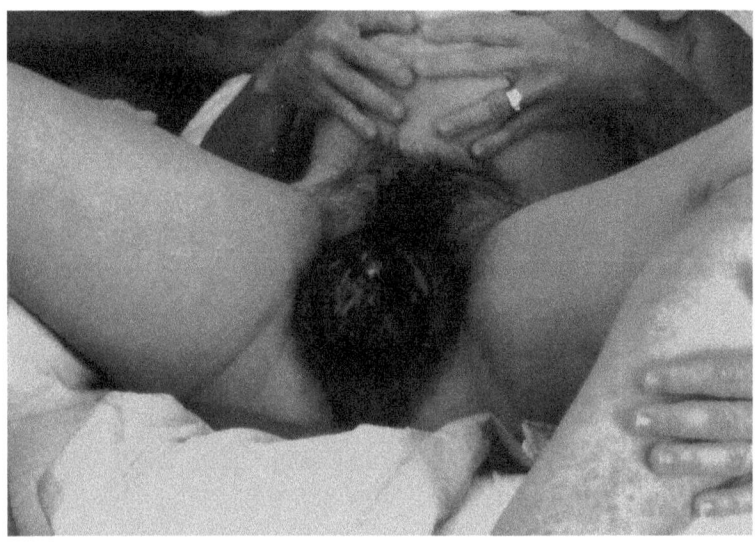

Baby's head has crowned, and is moving through the vagina

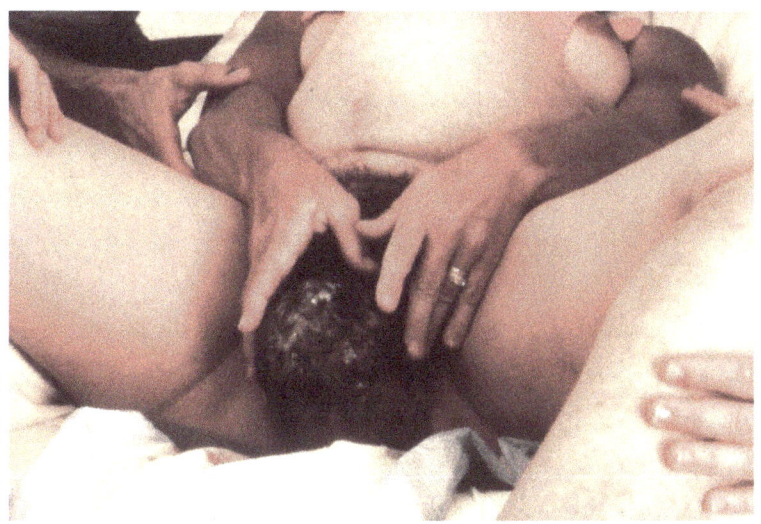

The mother touches the baby's head

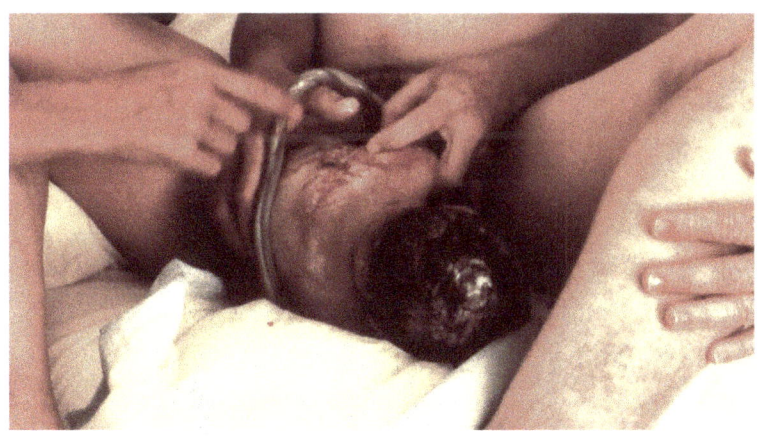

The baby is born

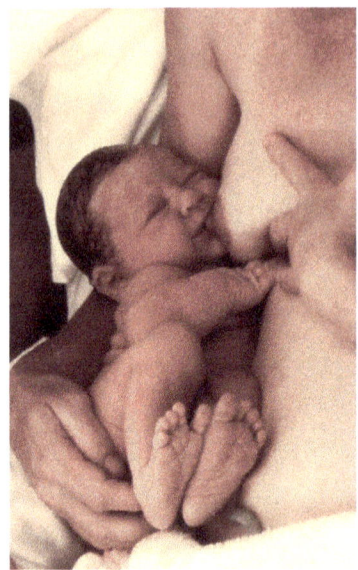

Newborn baby at the breast

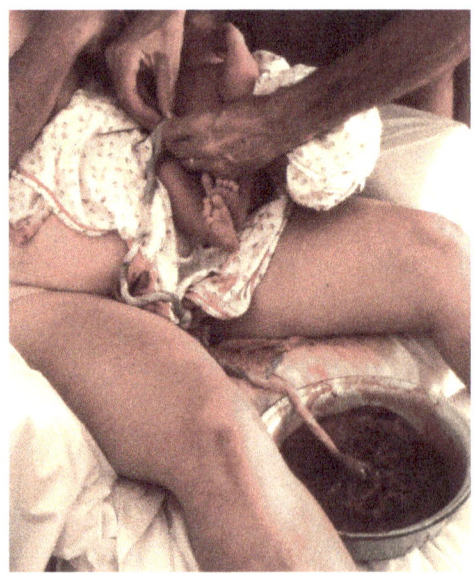

The Placenta and cutting the umbilical cord

## Chapter Seven — Homebirth

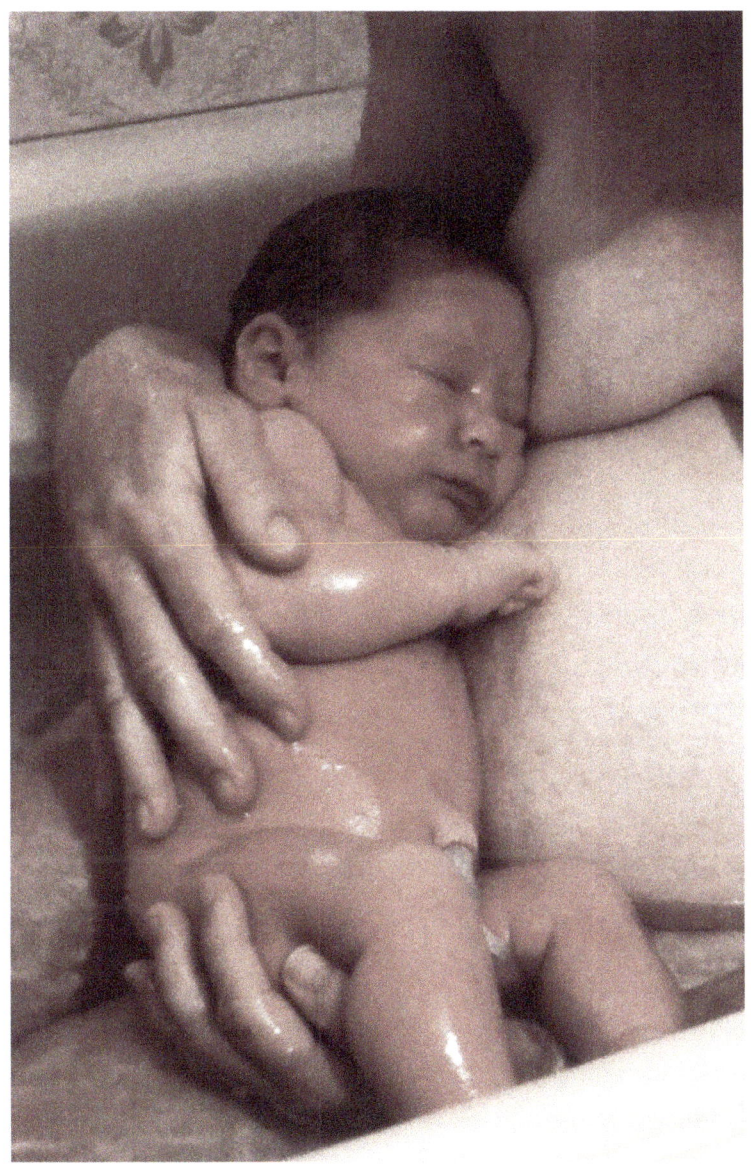

www.ingramcontent.com/pod-product-compliance
Lightning Source LLC
Chambersburg PA
CBHW062053290426
44109CB00027B/2815